Aissam Chibane

Surgery for digestive neuroendocrine neoplasia

Aissam Chibane

Surgery for digestive neuroendocrine neoplasia

ScienciaScripts

Cover image: www.ingimage.com

This book is a translation from the original published under ISBN 978-620-6-71595-5.

Publisher:
Sciencia Scripts
is a trademark of
Dodo Books Indian Ocean Ltd. and OmniScriptum S.R.L publishing group

120 High Road, East Finchley, London, N2 9ED, United Kingdom
Str. Armeneasca 28/1, office 1, Chisinau MD-2012, Republic of Moldova, Europe
Printed at: see last page
ISBN: 978-620-7-80066-7

Table of contents

Preamble

In this work, we wanted to keep a practical character even in the introduction of the problem and the literature review to shed light on the theoretical foundations of the subject.

We do not claim to exhaust the subject, nor to solve all the problems still posed by digestive neuroendocrine neoplasia.

This study in no way detracts from the interest of a resolutely technical presentation; on the other hand, it will remain useful for young medical students, even if it is offered to specialists.

In fact, we've had the courage to abandon the routine paradigms of the usual presentations, and while we've borrowed material from a profuse literature, we offer a rejuvenated description that takes into account the most recent references. This is particularly noticeable in the presentation of surgical indications and in the pages devoted to relative propositions or emphasis. The complex interplay of peculiarities is carefully examined, however brief it may be: a simple passage in the discussion chapter can initiate further research. At the same time, the sentences used as examples leave the reader free to criticize the analysis if he or she sees fit.

By studying the surgical aspects of neuroendocrine neoplasia, we have made a valuable contribution to enriching the Algiers Faculty of Medicine with this document, thus giving those working in this field a new medium to use and refer to.

I. Chapter 1: Introduction and theoretical foundations

I.1 HISTORY OF TNE :

"A history of international cooperation

In 1870, the German physician Heidenhain described cells in the intestine and named them chromaffin cells, due to their ability to turn brown when treated with chromic salts. In 1888, his fellow countryman Lu-Barsch (Fig. 1-a) probably described for the first time several small tumors in the ileum of 2 patients at autopsy (1). Later, the Russian physician Kultschitzky (figure 1-b) described them as acidophilic basigranular cells. These cells can be identified by staining with chromium and silver salts and are therefore called Enterochromaffin cells, referring to their affinity for silver salts(2).

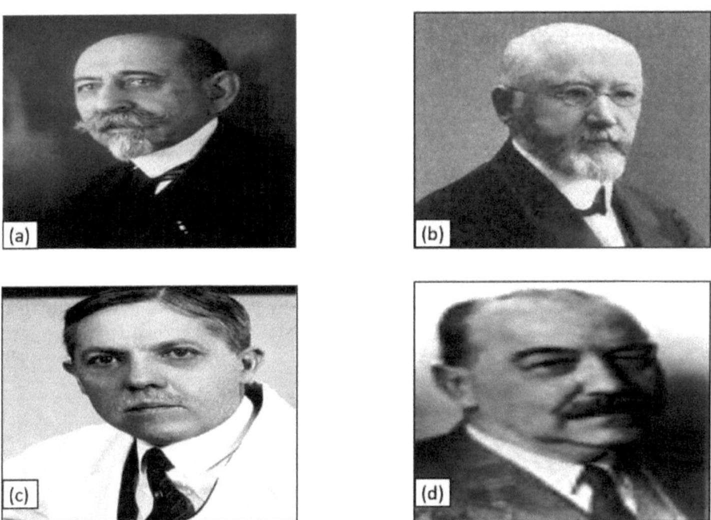

Figure 1: (a) Lubarsch, (b) Kultschitzky, (c) Masson and (d) Feyrter

In 1914, Pierre Masson (figure 1-c), a Canadian pathologist, showed that some of these cells were argentaffinous, capable of migrating from nerve plexuses, undergoing differentiation and secreting substances(3). In 1954, the Austrian pathologist Feyrter (fig. 1-d) isolated a diffuse cellular system whose elements are dispersed almost individually in the pancreatic excretory lining epithelium: a system with the value of an organ within an organ, each endowed with different functions (4).

The first large series of NNEs was described in 1961 by the American Moertel (figure 2-a), who reported 203 patients, with an incidence of 0.65% at autopsy. He also noted that these tumors more frequently localize distally along the small intestine, and that around 50% of 1-2 cm tumors metastasize (5). His classic 1987 article "An odyssey into the land of small tumors" updated this series, describing 183 patients who underwent surgical resection (6). Although 80% of patients were disease-free at 5 years, in long-term follow-up, up to 25 years, only 23% had not recurred. Moertel was also an early adopter of somatostatin analogues for symptomatic relief and chemotherapy for metastatic disease (7).

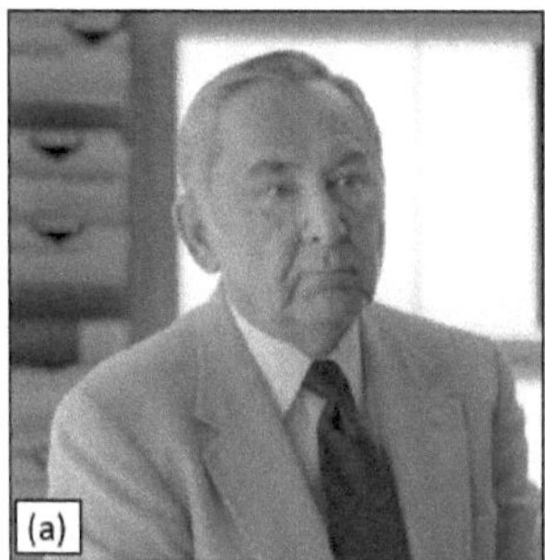

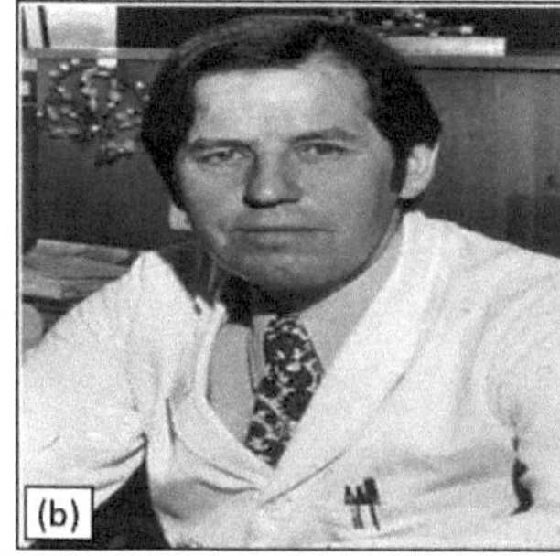

Figure 2: (a) Moertel & (b)Anthony Guy Everson

In 1966, British histologist Anthony Guy Everson (Figure 2-b) demonstrated that clear cells have particulate chemical properties (amine precursor uptake and decarboxylation) and grouped them together in a set called the APUD system (8).Today, we know that not all active endocrine cells take up amine, and so the name diffuse neuroendocrine system (DNS) is preferable.

I.2 INTRODUCTION :

Digestive neuroendocrine neoplasia (DNEN) is a highly heterogeneous group of tumors that develop from neuroendocrine cells of the digestive system. Neuroendocrine cells are specialized cells capable of producing hormones and/or neurotransmitters, and involved in the regulation of various physiological functions. NNE are classified according to their histological grade, tumor stage and secretory capacity. There are two main categories of NET: neuroendocrine tumors (NETs), which are well-differentiated, and neuroendocrine carcinomas (NECs), which are poorly differentiated. NETs are generally slow-growing and have a good prognosis, while NECs are fast-growing and have a poor prognosis. NNEs may be asymptomatic, or manifest as a mechanical mass syndrome or secretory syndromes linked to hormonal secretion. Diagnosis is based on imaging, biopsy and serum marker assays. Treatment depends on tumor type, location, stage and secretory activity. It may involve surgery, embolization, radiotherapy, chemotherapy, somatostatin analogues, targeted therapies or radio peptides (9,10).

I.3 THEORETICAL BACKGROUND :

The main function of the gastrointestinal tract is to deliver nutrients to our body via the processes of ingestion, motility, secretion, digestion and absorption; this occurs through a complex coordination of digestive processes that are regulated by the intrinsic endocrine and nervous systems. Although the nervous system exerts an influence on many digestive processes, the gastrointestinal tract is the largest endocrine organ in the human body and produces numerous mediators that play an essential role in regulating the functions of the gastrointestinal tract (11).

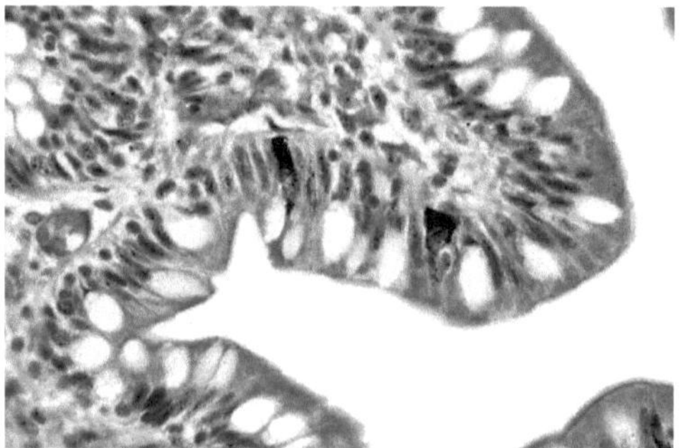

Figure 3: Intestinal villosity (12)

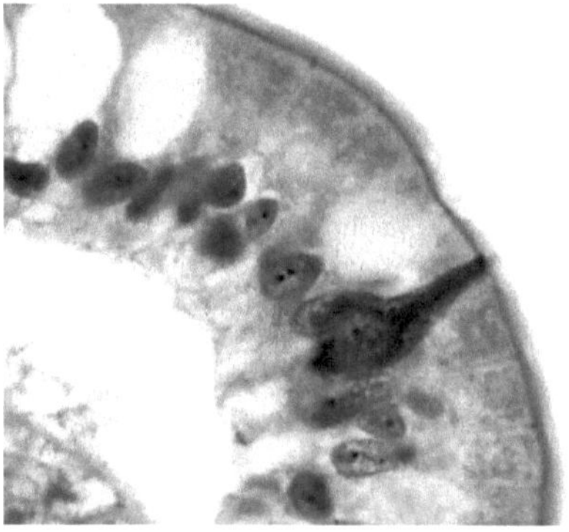

Figure 4: Silver cell (12)

I.3.1 Anatomy and physiology of the neuroendocrine system :

1.3.1.1 The CNN neuroendocrine cell:

A neuroendocrine cell (CNN) is a cell that receives neuronal input (neurotransmitters released by nerve cells or neurosecre trice cells) and, as a result of this input, releases message molecules (hor mones) into the bloodstream. Neuroendocrine cells are similar to neurons, but they also produce hormones in the same way as cells in the docrine system (endocrine cells). (11)

1.3.1.2 Gastrointestinal hormones:

Gastrointestinal hormones are classified as endocrine, paracrine or neurocrine, depending on how the molecule is delivered to its target cell(s). Endocrine hormones are secreted by en- terroendocrine cells directly into the bloodstream, passing from the portal circulation to the systemic circulation, before being delivered to target cells with the specificity of the hormone's receptor. The five gastrointestinal hormones described as endocrine are gastrin, cholecystokinin (CCK), secretin, glucose-dependent insulinotropic peptide (GIP) and motilin. Enteroendocrine cells also secrete paracrine hormones, but these diffuse into the extracellular space to act locally on target tissues and do not enter the systemic circulation. Two examples of paracrine hormones are somatostatin and histamine. In addition, some hormones can function via a combination of endocrine and paracrine mechanisms. These include glucagon-like peptide-1 (GLP-1), pancreatic polypeptide and peptide YY. Finally, neurocrine hormones are secreted by the non-cholinergic postganglionic neurons of the enteric nervous system. Three neurocrine hormones with important physiological functions in the gut are vasoactive intestinal peptide (VIP), gastrin-releasing peptide (GRP) and enkephalins(12).

1.3.1.3 Specialized enteroendocrine cells :

These gastrointestinal hormones are synthesized in the enteroendocrine cells of the gastrointestinal mucosa. These are specialized epithelial cells derived from endoderm stem cells located at the base of the intestinal crypts. These cells are dispersed throughout the gastrointestinal mucosa, distributed between epithelial cells from the eosophagus to the rectum. In addition, these enteroendocrine cells possess hormone-containing granules concentrated at the basolateral membrane, adjacent to the capillaries, which secrete their hormones by exocytosis in response to a wide range of stimuli related to food intake. These stimuli include small peptides, amino acids, fatty acids, oral glucose, organ distension and vagal stimulation (13).

G cells secrete gastrin in the antrum of the stomach and duodenum in response to the presence of degradation products of protein digestion (such as amino acids and small peptides), distension by feeding and stimulation of the vagus nerve by GRP. More specifically, phenylalanine and tryptophan are the most potent stimulators of gastrin secretion among the products of protein digestion(11). CCK is secreted by I-cells in the duodenum and jejunum in response to acids and monoglycerides (but not triglycerides), as well as to the presence of protein digestion products. Secretin is secreted by duodenal S cells in response to H+ and fatty acids in the lumen. Specifically, a pH below 4.5 signals the arrival of gastric contents, initiating the release of secretin. GIP is secreted by K-cells in the duodenum and jejunum in response to glucose, amino acids and fatty acids. GIP is the only gastrointestinal hormone to respond to all three types of macronutrient, and more recent studies suggest that changes in intraluminal osmolarity may be what stimulates GIP secretion (14).

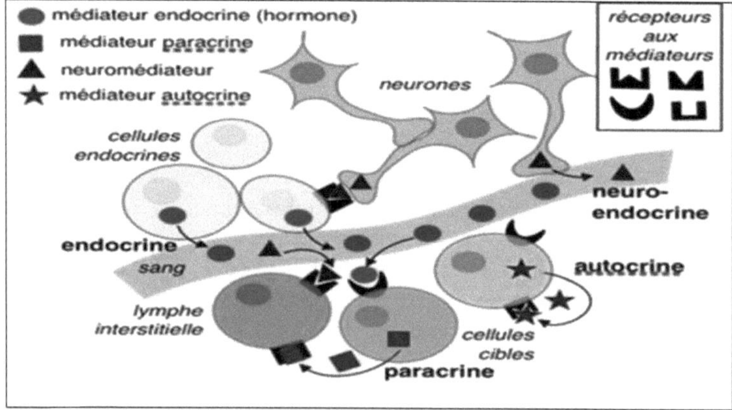

Figure 3: Neuroendocrine cell

I.3.1.4 Location of CNNs in the body :

Neuroendocrine cells are found throughout most of the body. They are mainly found scattered throughout the digestive tract (in the small intestine, rectum, stomach, colon, esophagus and appendix), gallbladder, pancreas (pancreatic islets) and thyroid (C cells). Neuroendocrine cells are also commonly found in the lungs or in the airways within the lungs (bronchi), as well as in the airways of the head and neck. The neuroendocrine cells scattered throughout these organs are often referred to as the diffuse neuroendocrine system. The pituitary gland, the parathyroid glands and the inner layer of the adrenal gland (medulla) are almost all composed of neuroendocrine cells. Other sites where neuroendocrine cells are found include the thymus, kidneys, liver, prostate, skin, cervix, ovaries and testes (15).

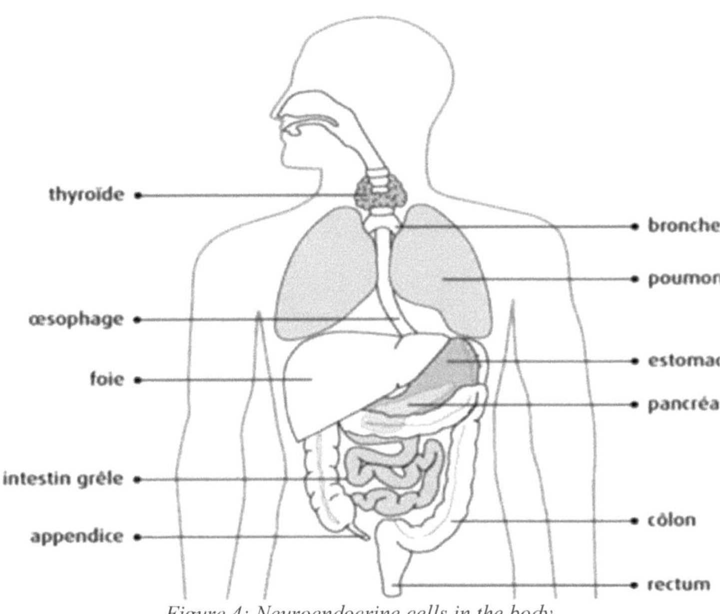

Figure 4: Neuroendocrine cells in the body

I.3.2 NNED classifications :

The classification of digestive NNE has evolved over the years to better reflect their clinical and biological heterogeneity. They are classified according to their anatomical origin, histological grade, differentiation and secretory capacity.

I.3.2.1 According to anatomical origin :

Digestive NNE is divided into two main groups: NNE of the gastroenteropancreatic (GEP) tract and NNE of the colon-rectum. NNEs of the GEP tract are the most common, accounting for around 70% of cases. They may be located in the stomach, duodenum, jejunum, ileum, appendix, pancreas or liver. Colon-rectal NNEs are less common, accounting for around 15% of cases. They are mainly located in the rectum, but can also involve the ascending, transverse or descending colon (16). This division has an embryological explanation, taking into account the embryonic origin of each segment of the digestive tract.

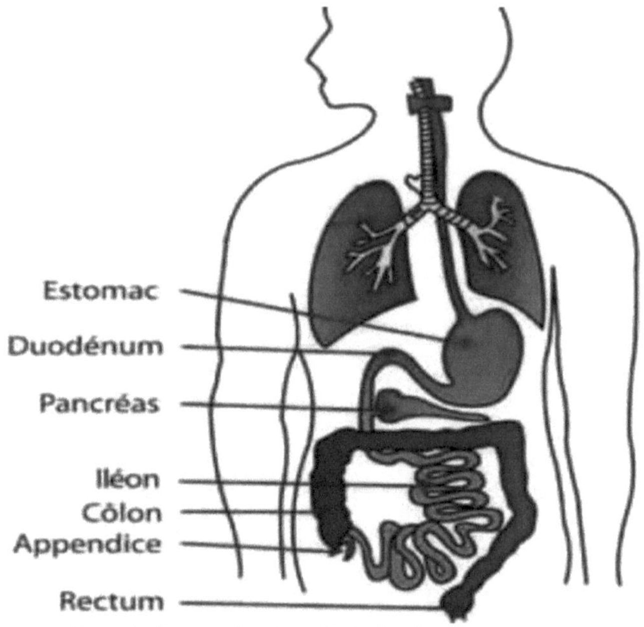

Figure 5: Neuroendocrine cells in the digestive tract

I.3.2.2 According to embryological origin :

Foregut foregut NNEs: develop from the primitive foregut, comprising the esophagus, stomach, proximal duodenum, proximal pancreas, upper respiratory tract and thyroid. Tumors in this category include bronchial, gastric, duodenal and pancreatic tumors. They tend to be well differentiated and may be associated with specific clinical syndromes, such as Zollinger-Ellison syndrome for gastric NETs and von Hippel-Lindau syndrome for pancreatic NETs (16).

Midgut NNE**:** arise from the primitive midgut, comprising the distal duodenum, ileum, jejunum, ascending and transverse colon, and appendix. Tumors in this category include appendicular, ileal and jejunal tumors. They are often less differentiated than Foregut NETs, but have a strong tendency to secrete hormones, leading to characteristic symptoms such as carcinoid syndrome (16).

Hindgut hindgut NETs: develop from the embryonic hindgut, comprising the descending colon, sigmoid colon, rectum, bladder, lower thyroid gland and lower parathyroid gland. This category includes distal and rectal colic.

They are often non-functional and may be less differentiated than Foregut NETs (17).

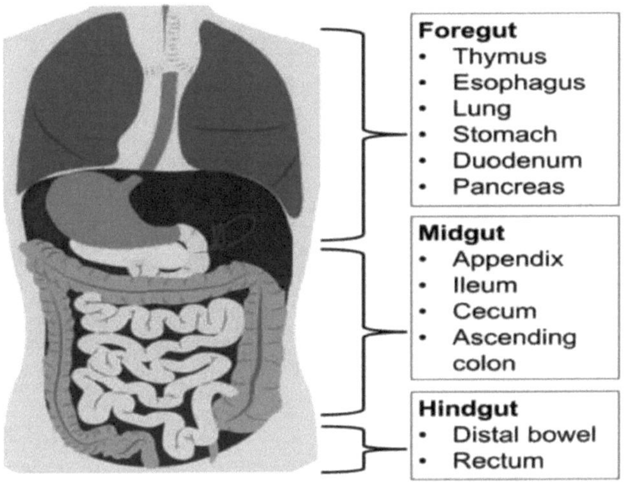

Figure 6: Embryological origin of NNEDs

I.3.2.3Differentiation :

1.3.2.3.1 Well-differentiated tumors :

Well-differentiated tumors include neuroendocrine tumors, which are generally of low grade and low aggressiveness. They are classified according to their histological grade, as described in the previous chapter, and also according to their anatomical location, notably the appendix, stomach, small intestine, colon and rectum (18).

1.3.2.3.2 Poorly differentiated tumors :

Poorly differentiated tumors, also known as neuroendocrine carcinomas, are more aggressive and tend to exhibit high cell proliferation. They are classified according to cellular component and nature as large- or small-cell carcinomas (18).

1.3.2.3.3 Mixed tumors :

Mixed tumors include well- or poorly-differentiated neuroendocrine components and another adenomatous or adenocarcinomatous contingent, which can complicate their classification and management (18).

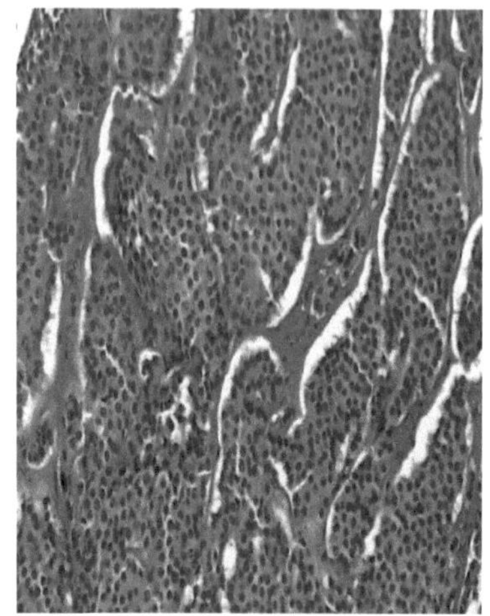

Figure 7:Well-differentiated NET (20)

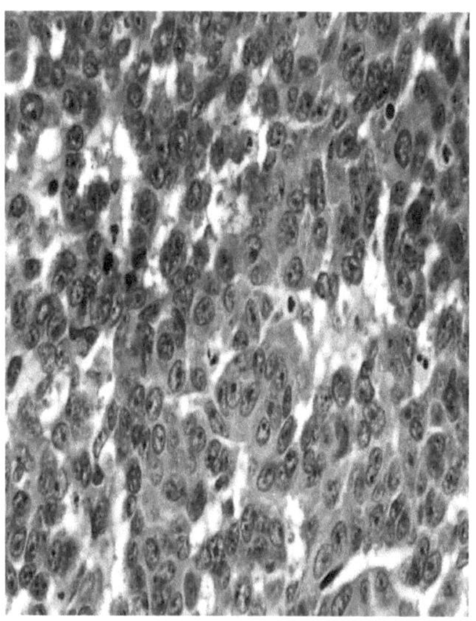

Figure 8: Poorly differentiated NET (20)

I.3.2.4 According to histological grade :

Digestive NNEs are classified according to the 2017 World Health

Organization (WHO) classification, which is being renewed in 2019, based on the rate of cell proliferation measured by the mitotic index or the percentage of cells expressing the Ki-67 protein. This classification distinguishes three grades: G1 (well-differentiated, low grade), G2 (well-differentiated, intermediate grade) and G3 (poorly differentiated, high grade). Histological grade is an important prognostic factor, influencing the choice of treatment and patient follow-up (18).

Table 1: Histopronostic classification of NNED (19)

	Ki67 (%)	Indice mitotique (mitoses pour 10 grands champs)
Grade 1	< 3	< 2
Grade 2	3-20	2-20
Grade 3	> 20	> 20

	Grade	Différenciation
Tumeur neuroendocrine G1	G 1	Bien différenciée
Tumeur neuroendocrine G2	G 2	Bien différenciée
Tumeur neuroendocrine G3	G 3	Bien différenciée
Carcinome neuroendocrine		Peu différenciée
Néoplasie mixte neuroendocrine - non neuroendocrine (MiNEN)	Tous grades	Association d'un contingent neuroendocrine et d'un contingent non-neuroendocrine

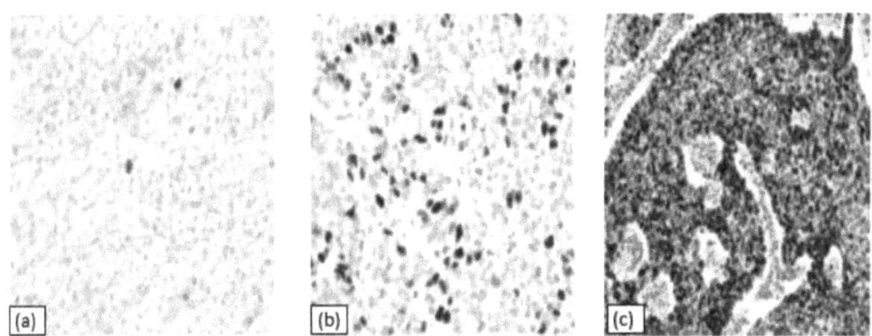

Figure 9:(a) TNEgrade 1, (b) TNEgrade 2, (c) TNEgrade 3

In 2022, the classification of digestive NNEs was updated by the WHO, retaining the same grading system as the previous one, with the introduction of a few modifications essentially concerning diagnostic, prognostic and theranostic biomarkers(20-22).Differential diagnosis between well-differentiated G3 NCTs and NECs is sometimes tricky; for this reason, the authors of this classification propose the use of immunohistochemical biomarkers likely to help distinguish between these two categories. These biomarkers include menin, DAXX and ATRX for the pancreas, and p53 and

Rb for other organs. When faced with inaugural NNE metastases with no known primary, the latest WHO classification proposes the use of certain transcription factors in IHC, which point to the origin of the primary, such as: TTF1 for pulmonary NNE; CDX2 and serotonin for intestinal NNE; PDX1, ISL1, DAXX/ATRX for pancreatic NNE (23). Pancytokeratins (CK); not limited to CK7 and CK20; usually rule out paraganglioma or pheochromocytoma in case of negativity. Some changes in terminology concerning small pancreatic lesions < 0.5 cm have been made by this new version; these were previously called "micro-adenomas" but the current classification advocates using the term "neuroendocrine microtumors" as these can give rise to lymph node metastases. Another concept has been updated: amphi-crine tumors have been excluded from the MINEN category (24).

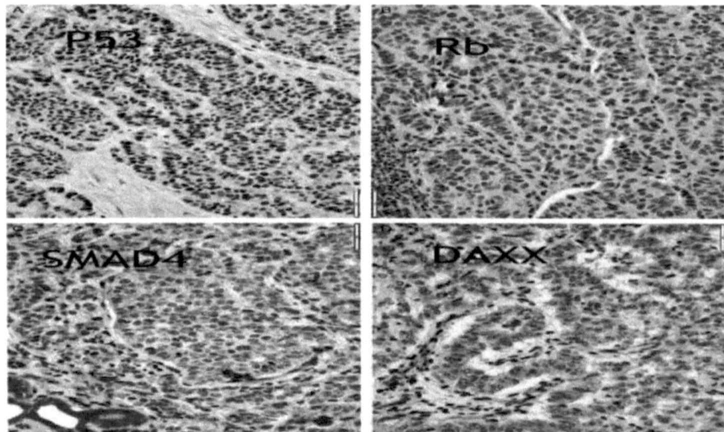

Figure 10: Distinguishing markers between CNE (top) and G3 NET (bottom)

I.3.2.5According to secreting power :

Digestive NNE are classified as either functional or non-functional. Functional NNE are those which produce clinical symptoms linked to excessive secretion of hormones or peptides by the tumor cells. Non-functional NNEs are those that do not produce specific hormonal symptoms, but may cause local or metastatic manifestations. Functional NETs are rarer than non-functional NETs, accounting for around 20% of cases (25). The most common clinical syndromes associated with functional NETs are carcinoid syndrome, Zollinger-Ellison syndrome, Verner-Morrison syndrome and insulinoma (17,26).

Table 2: Hormonal syndromes associated with pancreatic neuroendocrine tumors(19)

Hormone	Signes cliniques	Signes biologiques
Insuline	Tremblements, sueurs, palpitations, céphalées, confusion, flou visuel, amnésie, aggravation à jeun	↓ Glycémie ↑ Insulinémie ↑ Pro-insulinémie ↑ Peptide C
Gastrine	Ulcères et œsophagite peptiques, hémorragie digestive haute, diarrhée	↑ Gastrinémie à jeun ↑ Débit acide basal Test à la sécrétine
Glucagon	Diabète, érythème nécrolytique migrateur, diarrhée, perte de poids, phlébite, troubles visuels	↑ Glucagononémie ↑ Glycémie Anémie
Peptide vasointestinal	Douleurs abdominales diarrhée aqueuse, perte de poids, déshydratation	↑ VIP ↓ Kaliémie Acidose métabolique

I.3.2.6 According to molecular profile :

Recent advances in the molecular characterization of digestive NNE have led to a better understanding of their heterogeneity and the identification of new therapeutic targets. Molecular classifications aim to group tumors according to their genetic alterations, gene expression profiles and affected signaling pathways (18).

Genetic profile :

Some digestive NNEs have specific mutations, such as DNA methyl ethyl transferase 3A (DNMT3A) and isoniazid reactivity A (ARID1A) gene mutations, which can influence therapeutic response (18).

Genetic expression :

Gene expression analysis has identified NNE subgroups with distinct molecular signatures, which may also have prognostic and therapeutic implications (18).

Syndromic expression of predisposition :

Around 5% of gastroenteropancreatic NETs develop as part of an inherited genetic predisposition syndrome. The two most common syndromes are: multiple endocrine neoplasia type 1 (MEN1), associated with a broad spectrum of tumors including duodenopancreatic, thymic and bronchial NETs, and von Hippel-Lindau syndrome (VHL), associated with pancreatic NETs. Two other syndromes have a low incidence of NETs: neurofibromatosis type 1 (NF1), associated with duodenal somatostatinomas, and tuberous sclerosis of Bourneville (TSC), associated with pancreatic NETs. Two exceptional syndromes have a high incidence of NETs: multiple endocrine neoplasia type 4 (NEM4), whose tumor spectrum is similar to that of NEM1, and glucagon cell hyperplasia/neoplasia syndrome (GCHN), which is strictly pancreatic in expression. Other syndromes remain to be characterized, notably in the context of familial forms of intestinal NET. The diagnosis is evoked by the clinical context: onset at an early age, involvement of several organs, family history. With the exception of VHL and NF1, the tumours themselves do not usually present any particular anatomopathological characteristics; they are most often NETs of well-differentiated morphology and low histological grade, with a good prognosis, except for thymic lesions in NEM1. However, their association with endocrine and non-endocrine lesions of adjacent tissue is highly suggestive. The pathologist retains an important role not only in evoking the diagnosis in certain specific cases, but above all in contributing effectively to the management of these patients and their families, which is the responsibility of specialized centers (27).

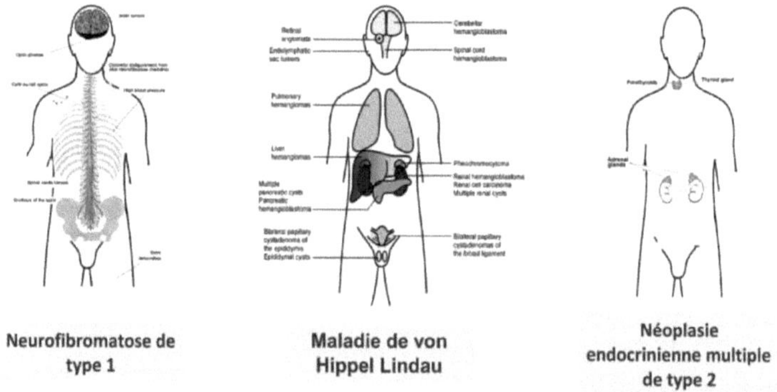

Figure 11: Schematic representation of the main syndromic EODs

Table 3: Syndromes and genes involved

Syndrome	Gene involved	Endocrine lesions
NEM 1	MEN 1	Pituitary adenomas
		Parathyroid adenomas
		Adrenocortical tumor
		Duodenopancreatic NETs
		Thymic NET
		Bronchial NETs
		Secondary gastric NETs
VHL syndrome	VHL	Paragangliomas/phaeochromocytomas
		Pancreatic NETs
Neurofibromatosis type 1	NF1	Paragangliomas/phaeochromocytomas
		Duodenal NET
Tuberous sclerosis of Bourneville NEM 4	TCS1-TCS2 CDKNIB	Pancreatic NETs
		Pituitary adenomas

		Parathyroid adenomas
Glucagon cell hyperplasia/neoplasia syndrome	GCGR	Pancreatic NETs
Familial forms of intestinal NETs	IMPK	Entero-chromaffin NETs of the small intestine

I.3.3 Epidemiology :

Neuroendocrine neoplasia (NEN) is a heterogeneous class of rare tumors, accounting for around 1% of digestive cancers and 2-3% of endocrine cancers (9). Since around two-thirds of NNEs arise in the gastroenteropancreatic system, which mainly comprises the stomach, small intestine, colon, appendix, rectum and pancreas, gastroenteropancreatic NNE (GEP-NNE) is the main subtype of NNE (28).

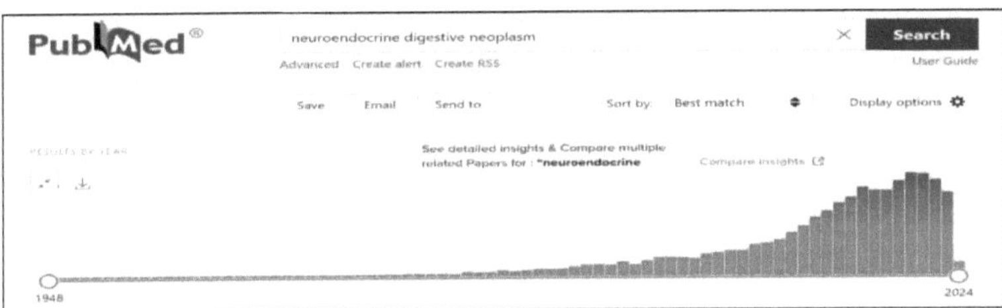

Figure 12: NNE search results on pub Med

The growing number of articles published each year on NNE is evidence that worldwide attention to NNE has increased, which may be due to the rise in reported incidence.

However, to our knowledge, there is a lack of up-to-date data on the epidemiological characteristics and survival analysis of patients with NNE-GEP. On the other hand, given the rarity of NNE-GEP, most studies on NNE-GEP are based on very small numbers and mo- nocentric studies. In addition, population-based studies have never specifically targeted NNE-GEP, but rather addressed NNE by organ (e.g., stomach, colon, small intestine, appendix, or pancreas).

I.3.3.1 Incidence:

The incidence of digestive NNE varies considerably according to anatomical location. NNE of the terminal ileum and appendix are among the most common, accounting for up to 67% of all digestive NNE, with an incidence rate varying from 0.2 to 2.7 cases per 100,000 people per year, depending on the region (25,29). NNE of the pancreas, although less frequent, is often more aggressive, with an incidence rate of 0.3 to 1.5 cases per 100,000 people per year (16,30).

1.3.3.2 Prevalence :

The prevalence of digestive NNE is rising steadily, mainly due to improved detection and prolonged patient survival. Global prevalence is estimated at around 35 cases per 100,000 people(31). NNE of the stomach and colon are among the most frequent, while NNE of the terminal ileum and pancreas are less frequent (16,32).

1.3.3.3 Geographical distribution :

There are significant geographical differences in the incidence of digestive NNE. For example, NNE of the stomach is more common in Asia, with incidence rates ranging from 0.11 to 0.74 cases per 100,000 people per year, while NNE of the terminal ileum is more common in Western Europe and North America, with rates of up to 1.74 cases per 100,000 people per year(33,34). These geographical variations can be attributed to environmental, genetic and dietary factors.

1.3.3.4 Potential Risk Factors :

Several potential risk factors have been identified in the epidemiology of digestive NNE:

Genetic factors: A family history of NNE and hereditary syndromes such as multiple endocrine neoplasia type 1 (MEN1) and von Hippel-Lindau syndrome (VHL) are associated with an increased risk.

Diet: Diets high in fat, red meat and alcohol have been linked to an increased risk of developing digestive NNE(35).

Toxin exposure: Exposure to carcinogens such as smoking and asbestos has been suggested as a risk factor for pulmonary NETs(36).

Emerging Trends :

Emerging trends in the epidemiology of digestive NNE include an increase in incidence, mainly due to greater awareness and improved diagnostic techniques. In addition, a growing understanding of the genetic basis of NNE has paved the way for more targeted therapeutic approaches and improved patient management.

1.3.3.5 Data in Algeria :

The rarity of the clinical presentation of these neoplasias and the lack of studies on the subject mean that we are deprived of epidemiological data in our country. Nevertheless, a dynamic is beginning to take shape around a core of experts who regularly organize RCP meetings with a database in the central region and in Oranie to collect data from all patients identified. A descriptive series in the Blida pathological anatomy department collected 128 cases, with an increase in the incidence of cases between 2020 (26 cases) and 2021 (33 cases) (24). Another series by Dr Khalifa in Oran studied 102 cases.

1.3.3.6 Data from the Maghreb :

To date, we have no data on the incidence of digestive NNE in neighboring Maghreb countries (Morocco and Tunisia).

Two retrospective Moroccan and Tunisian studies of 53 and 26 patients respectively report a mean age of 56 in the Moroccan series and 49 in the Tunisian series (24).

1.3.3.7 Data in Europe :

According to a recent study based on data from 76 registries covering 24 European countries, the worldwide population-standardized incidence of digestive NETs was 3.56 cases per 100,000 inhabitants per year between 1995 and 2012 (25,31). Incidence was higher in men than in women 4.13 vs. 3.02, and increased with age, peaking between 70 and 79. Incidence also varied by region, with the highest rates in Northern Europe 5.63 and the lowest in Eastern Europe 2.01. Incidence also differed according to digestive NNE subtype, with the highest rates for pancreatic NNE 1.32 and small intestine NNE 0.86, and the lowest for stomach NNE 0.29 and colon-rectum NNE 0.28 (31).

1.3.3.8 Data in the USA:

The population-based study using information from the National Cancer Institute's Surveillance, Epidemiology and End Results (SEER) program in the USA to systematically analyze the epidemiological, clinical and prognostic features of NNE-GEP is considered a benchmark of current epidemiological data worldwide. Due to the complex and inconsistent treatment of NNE-GEP, the prognosis of patients with NNE-GEP is still difficult to assess (37).

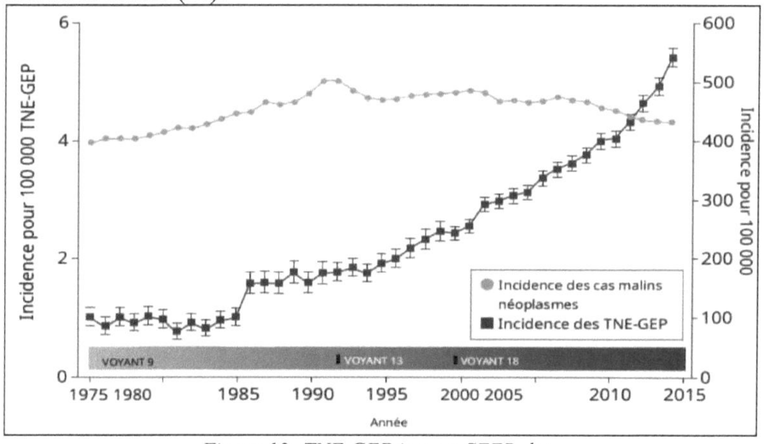

Figure 13: TNE GEP impact SEER data

In this study, the incidence and prevalence of NET-GEP continued to rise over 40 years, particularly in specific sites (such as the rectum and stomach) (37).

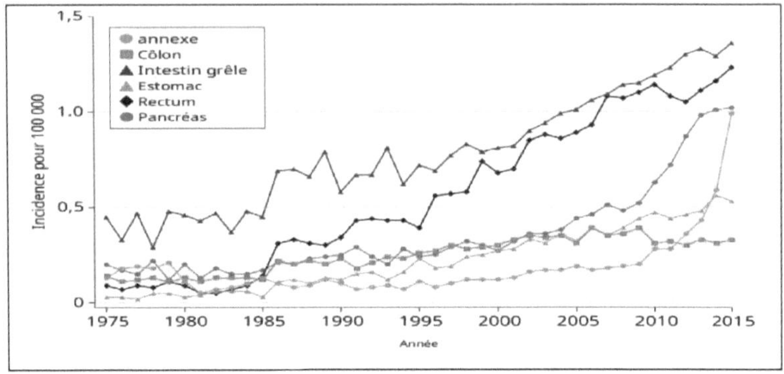

Figure 14: NNE incidence by organ

I.3.3.9 Data in Japan:

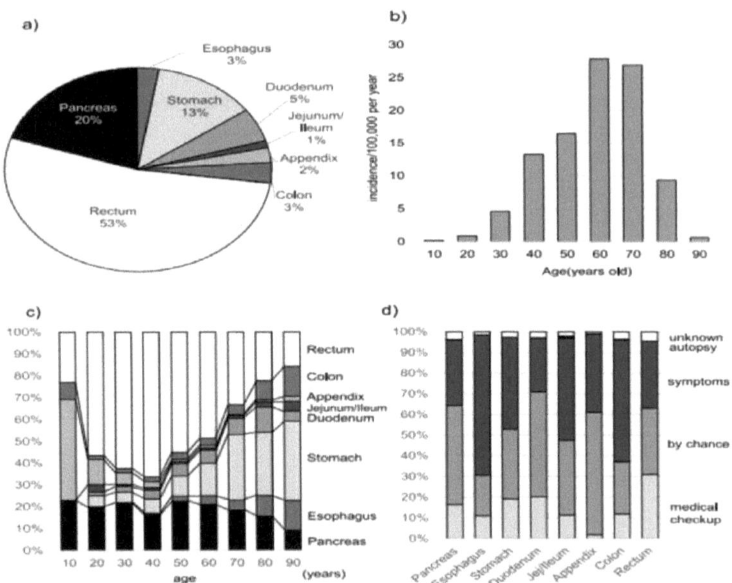

Figure 15: Epidemiological data in Japan

A population-based study using data from the Japanese National Cancer Registry (NCR) was conducted to evaluate patients with (NNE-GEP) in 2016. Associated population data were used to determine the age-adjusted annual rate. A total of 6,735 people were diagnosed with NNE GEP in Japan in 2016. The annual incidence was 0.70/100,000 inhabitants per year for pancreatic NNE and 2.84/100,000 inhabitants per year for gastrointestinal NNE. Ileal NEN accounted for only 1% of total GEP NEN in Japan. Most NENs in the oesophagus or lungs were neuroendocrine carcinomas (NECs), while the majority of those in the duodenum, ileum, appendix and rectum were grade 1 neuroendocrine tumours (NETs). The median age at initial diagnosis was between 60 and 65 years (38).

I.4 DIAGNOSIS AND PRE-OPERATIVE EVALUATION OF NNE-DIGESTIVES :

Digestive neuroendocrine neoplasia (DNEN) is a rare tumor, but early diagnosis is of vital importance for effective patient management. Diagnosis is based on a multidisciplinary approach, combining clinical, biological, morphological and functional data. The diagnostic approach comprises the following steps:

I.4.1 Clinical :

Questioning and clinical examination of the patient allow us to look for signs and symptoms suggestive of NNE, such as carcinoid syndrome, Zollinger-Ellison syndrome, Verner-Morrison syndrome, or local or metastatic manifestations of the tumor.
These signs are often inconstant and non-specific, which can complicate diagnosis. Common manifestations include:

1.4.1.1 Gastrointestinal symptoms :

Such as abdominal pain, diarrhea, constipation, gastrointestinal bleeding.

1.4.1.2 Hormonal symptoms :

Some digestive NNE secrete hormones, leading to flush-like symptoms such as hot flushes, flushing, erythema, hypoglycemia in the case of insulinoma, digestive disorders and fluctuations in blood pressure(39).

I.4.1.3 Obstructive symptoms :

Intestinal obstruction may occur as an emergency or subacutely as a result of tumor growth.
Early diagnosis is often based on a strong clinical suspicion combined with appropriate confirmatory tests.

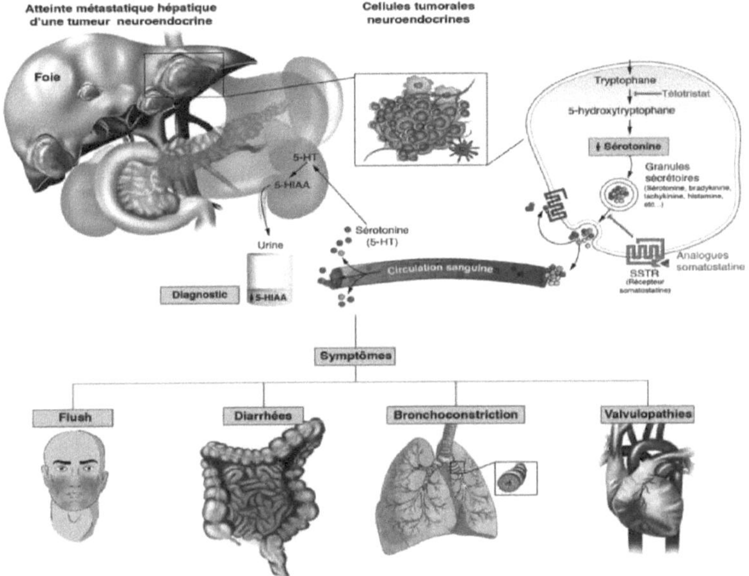

Figure 16: Consequences of secretion and symptoms of carcinoid syndrome

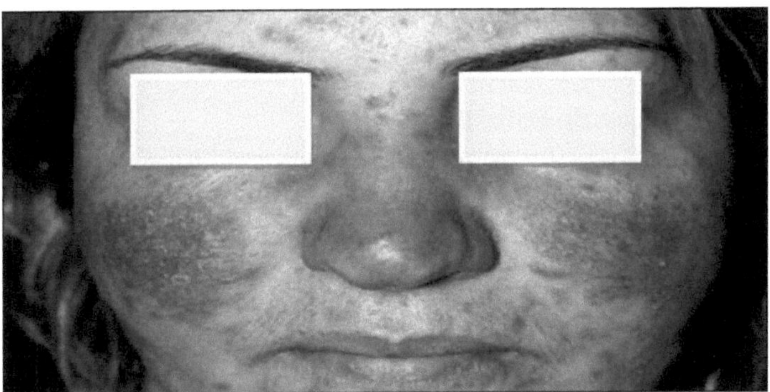

Figure 17: Facial erythema, a sign of flush impregnation

I.4.2 Organic :

By measuring serum tumor markers, which are substances produced by neuroendocrine cells or in response to their hormonal activity. The main markers are

1.4.2.1 Chromogranin A:

An increase in chromogranin A is often observed in NNE and can serve as a marker for follow-up (40).

Plasma CgA levels are sensitive and early NNE in relation to tumor burden and have been used to monitor treatment effects (4143). However, CgA levels are not specific as they are elevated with all types of NET and some non-endocrine malignancies (such as prostate carcinoma). CgA values are also increased due to endocrine cell hyperplasia in chronic atrophic gastritis (CAG) (elevated levels) and in patients with renal failure, liver failure, heart failure, stress and inflammatory bowel disease and due to chronic proton pump inhibitor (PPI) (moderately elevated values). However ,a decrease ≥ 80% predicts resolution of symptoms and stabilization of the disease (44).

1.4.2.2 The 5HIAA:

NNEs often produce excess serotonin, which is then metabolized to 5 HIAA. Excess HIAA is excreted in the urine, making it a potential biomarker for the diagnosis and monitoring of NNE. Elevated levels of the serotonin metabolite 5-hydroxyindoleacetic acid (5-HIAA) in 24-hour urine samples are specific markers in 85% of serotonin-producing NETs, but are only seen in advanced disease and usually signify the presence of liver metastases (42). The increase may be caused by tryptophan/serotonin-rich foods (bananas, avocados, plums, eggplants, chocolate, figs, tomatoes, pineapple, pecans, walnuts and wine), which should be avoided prior to urine sampling for 5 HIAA measurement (41,42). A reduction in urinary 5-HIAA concentrations of 80% or more (or normalization) was predictive of symptomatic relief but not of disease stabilization (45).

1.4.2.3 Specific hormones :

Blood levels of specific hormones, such as gastrin, insulin, glucagon, serotonin and histamine, can be measured to confirm hormone secretion.

1.4.2.4 Progastrin-Releasing Peptide (ProGRP):

This marker can be used, but not for digestive NNE; it is recommended for pulmonary NNE with high neurosecretion.

1.4.2.5 Genomics :

Measurement of serum biomarkers, such as chromogranin A and serotonin, remains an important screening and follow-up tool for NETs. In addition, the study of NET genomics has revealed specific molecular alterations, such as mutations in MEN1, DAXX, and ATRX, which have prognostic and therapeutic implications (46,47).

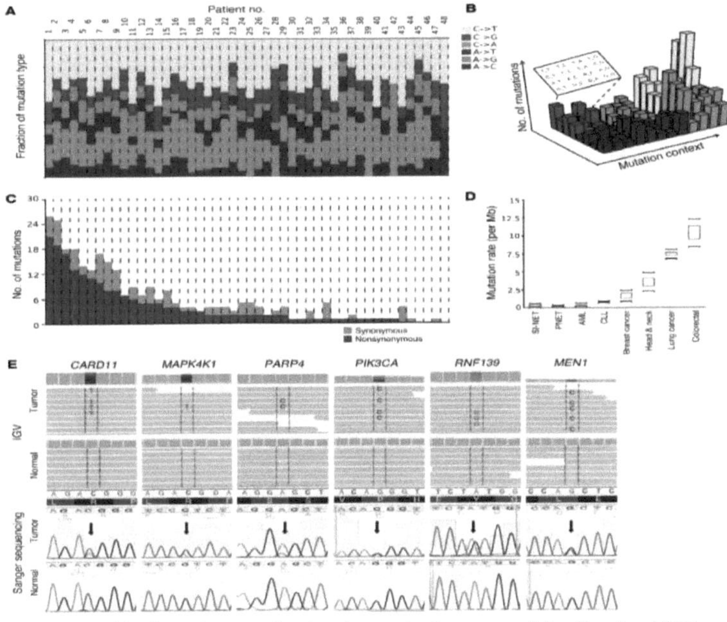

Figure 18: Somatic mutation landscape in the genes of the Grecian NNE.

I.4.3 Radiological :

The crucial contribution of medical imaging in the management of digestive neuroendocrine neoplasia is undeniable, with the aim of detecting, characterizing, staging and monitoring these rare and heterogeneous tumors. Imaging of digestive NNE is based on two types of technique: morphological imaging (ultrasound, CT and magnetic resonance) and functional imaging (scintigraphy and positron emission tomography).

I.4.3.1 Morphological imaging :

1.4.3.1.1 Ultrasound :

Ultrasound is often used as the first imaging test to evaluate liver and pancreatic lesions. It is non-invasive, widely available, and can help detect primary or metastatic lesions.

1.4.3.1.2 Computed tomography (CT) :

CT is essential for characterizing NEDs. It offers excellent spatial resolution and enables precise visualization of tumor size, location and vascularization (48).

1.4.3.1.3 Magnetic Resonance Imaging (MRI) :

MRI offers excellent tissue resolution and is particularly useful for pancreatic NNE, where it can distinguish benign from malignant lesions thanks to advanced sequences, such as diffusion and perfusion (49).

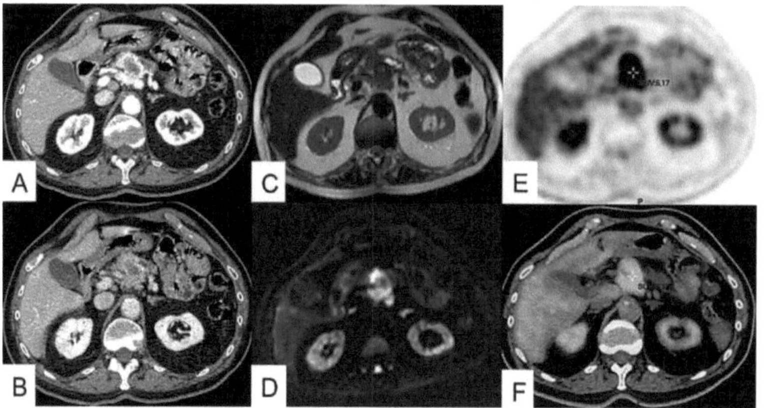

Figure 19: Radiological appearance of a pancreatic NET: AB CT, CD MRI, EFPETCT

I.4.3.2 Metabolic imaging :

1.4.3.2.1 Somatostatin scintigraphy:

Somatostatin scintigraphy or octreoscanner, using radiopharmaceuticals such as Indium-111 octreotide, is a method of choice for detecting well-differentiated NNEs expressing somatostatin receptors. It allows localization of primary tumors and metastases (50).

1.4.3.2.2 Somatostatin Positron Emission Tomography (PET):

Somatostatin PET, using radiopharmaceuticals such as 68Ga- DOTATATE, offers greater sensitivity and specificity than conventional somatostatin scintigraphy (octreoscan). It is particularly useful for imaging disease extension and monitoring response to treatment (51).

1.4.3.2.3 Fluorodeoxyglucose (FDG) PET :

FDG-PET can be used for poorly differentiated NNE or NNE with high metabolic activity. It can detect lesions with high glycolytic activity, often associated with more aggressive behavior (52).

Morphological and metabolic imaging play a crucial role in the management of digestive neuroendocrine neoplasia. Morphological imaging techniques such as ultrasound, CT and MRI enable precise characterization of lesions, while metabolic imaging, including somatostatin scintigraphy and PET, enables tumor detection, evaluation of extension and monitoring of response to treatment. The integration of these advanced imaging modalities into clinical practice is helping to improve the management of patients with NED.

I.4.3.3Imaging and staging :

CT plays a key role in the assessment of locoregional extension and distant metastases, particularly for NNE of the pancreas and gastrointestinal tract(53). MRI is useful for assessing liver metastases. Advanced techniques, such as diffusion and perfusion, can help characterize liver lesions;somatostatin PET (68Ga-DOTATAT)is also used for staging because of its high sensitivity for detecting lymph node and distant metastases(54).

I.4.3 Staging of digestive NNE :

NNEDs present diagnostic and therapeutic challenges. Accurate staging of NNEDs is essential to guide clinical management, determine prognosis and direct therapeutic decisions. Two reference classifications are commonly used for staging NNEDs: the Union Internationale Contre le Cancer (UICC) TNM classification and the European Neuroendocrine Tumor Society (ENETS) classification.

1.4.4.1 The UICC TNM Classification:

The most recent and most widely used in the world, it is a universally recognized system for staging cancers, including NNEDs. This classification is based on three main criteria:

1.4.4.1.1.1 T (Primary tumor)

This category assesses tumor size and local extension. Tumor size is an important prognostic factor for NEDs, with smaller tumors associated with a better prognosis (55).

1.4.4.1.1.2 N (regional lymph nodes)

Involvement of regional lymph nodes is assessed to determine the extent of disease in the region. Lymph node involvement is a significant prognostic indicator (56).

1.4.4.1.1.3 M (distant metastases) :

The presence of distant metastases indicates systemic disease progression. Metastases, particularly liver metastases, are common in NED patients and have a major impact on prognosis(46).

1.4.4.2 The ENETS Classification :

The oldest and most specific NNED. It was developed in 2006 and applies to NNEDs of the stomach, small intestine, colon-rectum and pancreas, taking into account histological and functional aspects, in addition to the criteria of the TNM classification. This classification is based on the following criteria:

I.4.4.2.1 G (Differentiation Grade) :

The histological grade of NNED varies from well-differentiated (G1, G2 and G3) to poorly differentiated (CNE). Grade is a major prognostic factor, influencing choice of treatment and long-term prognosis (57).

1.4.4.2.2 S (Primary Tumor Site) :

ENETS distinguishes NNEDs according to their primary site, such as pancreatic, intestinal, gastric, etc. Each site may have specific clinical and prognostic features. Each site may have specific clinical and prognostic features (58).

1.4.4.2.3 N (regional lymph nodes) :

Lymph node involvement is assessed in the ENETS classification, as in the TNM classification.

I.4.4.2.4 M (distant metastases) :

The presence of distant metastases is also taken into account in the ENETS classification.

8ème classification *Tumor-Node-Metastases* (TNM) des TNE selon l'UICC (2017). A noter que les CNE doivent être classés comme pour les carcinomes exocrines de localisation identique

	Estomac	Duodénum, ampoule	Pancréas	Intestin grêle	Appendice*	Côlon, rectum
TX	La tumeur primitive ne peut pas être évaluée					
T0	Pas de signe de tumeur primitive					
T1	Envahit la lamina propria ou la sous-muqueuse et ≤ 1 cm	Duodénum : Envahit la muqueuse ou la sous-muqueuse et ≤ 1 cm Ampoule : Confinée au sphincter d'Oddi et ≤ 1 cm	Limitée au pancréas et < 2 cm	Envahit la lamina propria ou la sous-muqueuse et ≤ 1 cm	Taille tumorale < 2 cm	Envahit la lamina propria ou la sous-muqueuse T1a : taille < 1 cm T1b : taille 1-2 cm
T2	Envahit la musculeuse ou > 1 cm	Duodénum : Envahit la musculeuse ou > 1 cm Ampoule : Envahit la sous-muqueuse ou la musculeuse duodénale ou > 1 cm	Limitée au pancréas et 2-4 cm	Envahit la musculeuse ou > 1 cm	Taille tumorale 2-4 cm	Envahit la musculeuse ou > 2 cm
T3	Envahit la sous-séreuse sans envahir la séreuse	Envahit le pancréas ou le tissu adipeux péri-pancréatique	Limitée au pancréas et > 4 cm, or envahit le duodénum ou la voie biliaire principale	Envahit la sous-séreuse sans envahir la séreuse	Taille tumorale > 4 cm ou envahit la sous-séreuse ou le méso-appendice	Envahit la sous-séreuse sans envahir la séreuse
T4	Envahit la séreuse ou les organes adjacents	Envahit la séreuse ou les autres organes adjacents	Envahit les organes adjacents ou la paroi des gros vaisseaux (tronc coeliaque, artère mésentérique supérieure)	Envahit la séreuse ou les organes adjacents	Envahit la séreuse ou les organes adjacents (sauf invasion pariétale de la sous-séreuse ou de l'intestin)	Envahit la séreuse ou les organes adjacents
NX	Les ganglions régionaux ne peuvent pas être évalués					
N0	Pas de signe de métastase ganglionnaire					
N1	Métastases ganglionnaires régionales			< 12 métastases ganglionnaires régionales	Métastases ganglionnaires régionales	
N2	-	-	-	> 12 métastases ganglionnaires régionales Ou large masse mésentérique (> 2 cm)	-	-
Mx	Les métastases à distance ne peuvent pas être évaluées					
M0	Pas de métastase à distance					
M1	Métastases à distance M1a : métastases hépatiques uniquement M1b : métastases disséminées à au moins une localisation extra-hépatique M1c : métastases hépatiques et extra-hépatiques					

* *Voir la section 11.3.2.6 concernant la classification TNM des TNE de l'appendice*

Figure 20: TNMs according to the TNCD NNE thesaurus of 7/11/2023 (58)

I.5 NNED surgery

I.5.1 Curative and palliative approaches :

Surgery plays a central role in the management of NNE-D, offering curative and palliative options with prospects of cure in early stages and palliative symptom relief in advanced stages.

I.5.1.1Curative surgical treatment

NNE-D detected at an early stage, generally limited to the mucosa or submucosa, is a candidate for curative surgical resection. The aim is to achieve en bloc resection with safe margins, while preserving organ function. Laparoscopy and robot-assisted surgery have expanded the possibilities for minimally invasive resections, enabling faster recovery and improved quality of life for patients, but remain controversial to this day (59).
Selection of patients for curative surgery depends on several factors, including tumor size and location, presence of lymph node metastases and histological grade. Thorough preoperative evaluation is essential to determine the extent of resection required (60).

I.5.1.2Palliative surgical treatment

For patients with advanced NNED with distant metastases or extensive local infiltration, palliative surgery can play a crucial role in symptom control and quality of life. Palliative interventions are primarily aimed at relieving bowel obstruction, controlling bleeding or reducing the effects of secretory syndrome. Intestinal bypass, partial tumor resection or tumor mass reduction may be performed to relieve obstruction. Selective embolization of tumor blood vessels or radiofrequency ablation are effective palliative approaches to control symptoms associated with peptide secretion.
Recent advances in imaging, such as mul- tiphasic contrast CT and somatostatin receptor scintigraphy, have enabled better preoperative assessment of advanced NNE-D, facilitating the planning of palliative interventions.

I.5.2 Radical and conservative approaches

Surgical techniques can be divided into two categories:

1.5.2.1 Conservative techniques :

Parenchyma sparing, aimed at preserving as much parenchyma as possible and preserving the functionality of the organs concerned.

1.5.2.2 Radical techniques

Involve more extensive resection with excision of regional lymph nodes. Conservative techniques are reserved for small (<2 cm), well-differentiated, non-functional NNEDs with no lymph node involvement. Radical techniques are indicated for large (>2 cm), poorly differentiated, functional or node-positive NEDs.

I.6 Surgical indications :

Surgery, the only curative treatment for well-differentiated localized neuroendocrine tumors, plays a major role in therapeutic strategy (61). It also has a place in metastatic forms. Whenever possible, surgery for liver metastases is recommended. This excision must be as complete as possible, at an acceptable operative risk. It should be supported by other complementary techniques such as preoperative embolization and radiofrequency (62). Two-stage hepatectomies can be used to treat all metastases (63).Hormone therapy with somatostatin analogues is of great importance for symptom control; particular caution must be exercised both before and during surgery. A multidisciplinary approach is essential to provide personalized therapy for patients with NNE. Clinical research and specialization in this field should be further encouraged. The natural history of gastro-entero-pancreatic neuroendocrine neoplasia (GEP) is becoming better understood, which explains the currently selective nature of surgical indications. Surgical resection, but also endoscopic resection and surveillance, can be proposed for gastric NETs, depending on their presentation, size and grade. In the case of NETs of the small intestine, digestive resection is often necessary, but it must be the best compromise between radical resection and functional outcome. Appendicular NETs are usually diagnosed on an emergency appendectomy specimen, but patients at high risk of lymph node metastasis and recurrence should be reoperated for radical resection. Rectal NETs are often diagnosed incidentally: the smallest (< 1 cm) can be resected endoscopically, but the most aggressive require radical proctectomy. Pancreatic NNE constitute a very broad spectrum, ranging from completely benign to highly aggressive tumors. Insulinomas are predominantly benign, but cause very disabling symptoms despite medical treatment, and should ideally be operated on by parenchymal-preserving resection, mainly by enucleation. Conversely, the symptoms of gastrinomas are effectively treated medically, but their resection requires a carcinological procedure. Non-functioning pancreatic NNEs are increasingly diagnosed as incidental findings. Depending on their size, presentation and patient characteristics, they justify resection (carcinological or parenchymal-preserving), or close monitoring.

1.6.1 Esophageal NNE :

They are very rare, <1% of all NNEs, and occur with a male predominance around the age of 60 (28,64). although the incidence is increasing on anatomopathological examinations of surgical specimens. Most tumours are neuroendocrine carcinomas with a very high Ki 67 and proliferation index, and metastases at the time of diagnosis (65,66). Tumors should only be operated on if radical resection is possible (64). In such cases, patients should undergo radical surgery with lymph node dissection.

1.6.2 Gastric NNE :

WHO guidelines describe three groups of gastric NETs derived from Enterochromaffin-like (ECL) cells: type 1, type 2 and type 3 (67). The majority of gastric NETs, type 1 (70-80%), occur in patients with hypergastrinemia due to chronic atrophic gastritis (GAC). Type 2 patients (5-8%) also present with hypergastrinemia, but due to Zollinger-Ellison syndrome (ZES) as part of a familial multiple endocrine neoplasia type 1 (MEN1) syndrome. Type 3 gastric NETs (15-20%) occur sporadically as solitary lesions in patients without hypergastrinemia; rare tumors may be of the non-ECL type. Important predictors of gastric NETs are size, type and histology. Neuroendocrine carcinomas of the stomach are very rare and have been termed type 4 (68).

Table 4: Summary of gastric NNEs

	TNE			CNE Type 4
	Type 1	**Type 2**	**Type 3**	
Relative frequency	70-80%	5-6 %	14-25%	6-8%
Aspect	<10 mm multiple	<10 mm multiple	Single svt >20 mm	Single svt >20 mm
Related pathology	Biermer anemia	SZE and NEM 1	no	No
Anapath	**Bien diff G 1**	**Bien diff G 1**	**Bien diff G 1, G 2**	**Little diff**
Gastrinemie	**Very high**	**Very high**	Normal	Normal
Metastases	<10 %	10-30%	**50-100%**	**80-100%**
Death/tumor	**no**	**<10%**	**25-30%**	**>50 %**

I.6.2.1 Type 1 gastric NETs :

Type 1 NETs occur with a female predominance (sex ratio 0.33) at an average age of around 65 years (41,64). Tumors arise in patients with chronic atrophic gastritis (GAC) with hypo or achlorhydria due to destruction of acid-secreting parietal cells. GAC may or may not be autoimmune (69). Hypergastrinemia occurs because gastrin-secreting G cells in the antrum are not inhibited in the absence of gastric acid. Excessive gastrin secretion, combined with other predisposing factors such as diet or possibly bacteria, will further stimulate ECL cell hyperplasia and the development of ECL cell tumors. Hyper-gastrinemia alone does not appear to cause gastric NETs, because tumors occur in a minority of patients with GAC and are not due to chronic PPI therapy or vagotomy (69-71). More than half of patients have vitamin B12 malabsorption and pernicious anemia, and in this population, NETs have often been revealed incidentally by endoscopy, as patients are usually asymptomatic. Although GAC is common in the elderly, only a few patients (1%) with markedly elevated serum gastrin values over a long period develop gastric NETs. NETs usually present as small multiple polyps (60%) in the gastric body and fundus or in the transition zone to the antrum, developing in a surrounding atrophic mucosa where ECL cell hyperplasia and dysplasia can be detected. Single tumors may present as extensive, round polypoid lesions; some may be flat and large, or appear as discolored patches or slight mucosal protrusions. The number and size vary from innumerable pin-sized lesions to a few prominent lesions measuring up to 1 to 1.5 cm and rarely up to 2 cm or more (69,70). Some are solitary and may be difficult to distinguish from adenopolyps, also present in patients with GAC. Only rare larger lesions may be ulcerated or bleeding. Small type 1 gastric NETs are benign, with low proliferation (grade 1) and a low risk of invasion beyond the submucosa. Larger lesions (> 1 cm) are also predominantly benign, but may occasionally invade the muscularis propria (< 10%) or have a higher grade. The incidence of regional lymph node metastases is low (<2-5%), distant liver metastases are exceptional (<2%) and disease-related deaths are rare, although earlier reports of a greater proportion of larger lesions described more frequent metastases (64,69,70). Exceptionally patients with GAC have had large invasive tumors, representing MINEN with poorly differentiated carcinomas and adenocarcinomas with poor prognosis.

I.6.2.2 Type 2 gastric NETs :

ECL cell hyperplasia can be detected in 80% of MEN1 patients with ZES, and 5-30% of MEN1-ZES patients develop type 2 gastric NETs (66,71-73). Patients have elevated gastric acid secretion and show a typical increase in mucosal thickness in contrast to the distinct atrophy of type 1 lesions. Patients with sporadic ZES may also often present with ECL cell hyperplasia, but rarely (<1%) develop gastric NETs. Type 2 gastric NETs occur in the gastric body and fundus, and occasionally in the antrum (72). They are also often multiple and usually small (<1 to 2 cm), but usually larger than type 1 tumors, and sometimes significantly larger, reaching 4 to 5 cm or more. Biopsies of the surrounding gastric mucosa show hypertrophy rather than atrophy. Tumor grade may be 1 or 2, and malignant potential is intermediate between GAC-associated and sporadic gastric NETs. Lymph node metastases occur in around 30% of patients, and liver metastases in 10-

20% (72). More aggressive tumours with liver metastases and higher grades have been more frequent with long-standing ZES. Poorly differentiated gastric NECs with local invasion, angioinvasion and high proliferation rates have sometimes been associated with MEN1.

I.6.2.3 Sporadic gastric TNT type 3 :

Sporadic type 3 gastric NETs occur in patients with normal serum gastrin. The tumors are more common in men, with a mean age of around 50 years (64,69-72). Calcemia and family history help exclude NEM1. The majority of patients present with symptoms similar to those of gastric adenocarcinoma, accompanied by pain, weight loss and gastrointestinal bleeding. The majority of type 3 NETs arise in the gastric body and fundus as solitary and often large tumors, usually > 2 cm; occasional tumors occur in the antral or prepyloric region (64,6972) . Tumours develop in the non-atrophic gastric mucosa, without ECL cell proliferation. Rare forms usually appearing in the antrum may originate from G cells (gastrin) or constitute a mixture of EC cells (serotonin) and other cell types, and may therefore be associated with a poorer prognosis. Most G-cell tumors show sparse gastrin staining. Tumors with intense gastrin reactivity are rare in the stomach, but can occur in the pre-pyloric mucosa and represent an exceptional cause of hypergastrinemia and ZES. Two-thirds of type 3 tumours infiltrate the muscular layer, and 50% invade all layers of the gastric wall. Regional lymph node metastases may be present in 20-50%, also in small tumors, and liver metastases eventually develop in two-thirds of patients (72) Sporadic gastric NETs may have an atypical histology, with pleomorphism, high mitosis rate and elevated Ki-67 index. Atypical tumours are larger, averaging around 5 cm in size, more frequently invasive and have a poor survival record(72).

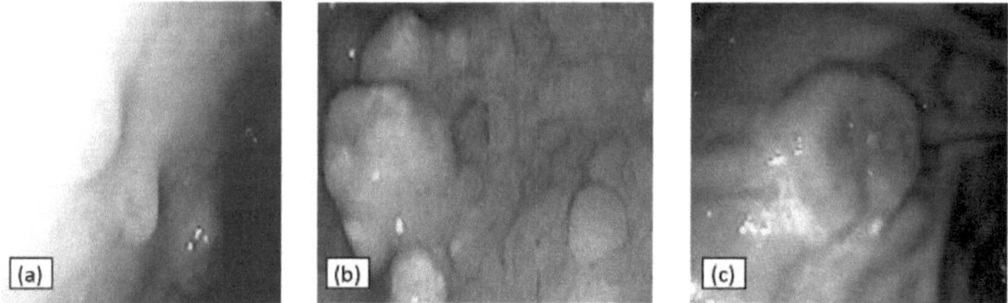

Figure 21 Gastric NNE on endoscopy (a) TNE type 1, (b) TNE type 2, (c) TNE type 3

I.6.2.4Gastric CNE "type 4 tumors" :

Gastric NNE type 4 is a more recently defined type, which is the rarest subtype. They do not originate from ECL cells and their growth is independent of gastrin. Most often, the lesion presents as a large polypoid lesion located anywhere in the stomach. Type 4 g -NENs are aggressive tumours with a high potential for invasion and metastasis (73).

I.6.3 Grecian NNE :

NNEG small bowel NETs, long referred to as "classic" midgut carcinoids, originate from intestinal enterochromaffin (EC) cells located in the intestinal crypts and can be recognized by the serotonergic immunoreactivity typical of tumor cells. Carcinoids can be detected in up to 1/150 of routine autopsies, indicating that tumors may remain silent throughout life (74).

They are mostly ileal, low-grade (G1, low G2), associated with mesenteric lymph node metastases (responsible for retractile mesenteritis in 20% of cases at diagnosis), metastatic to the liver (40%) and may be revealed by intestinal obstructions (20%) (75-77). Mesenteric extension is responsible for vascular engraftment, so that complete resection of the tumor (possibly including the right colon) may result in extensive resection with risk of secondary short bowel syndrome. The extent of mesenteric resection must be determined to achieve the best compromise between radical surgery and postoperative functional impairment. Complete resection of the tumour results in a survival rate of 75% to 85% at 5 years, but follow-up must be extended to at least 10 years due to the very slow natural evolution of these tumours.

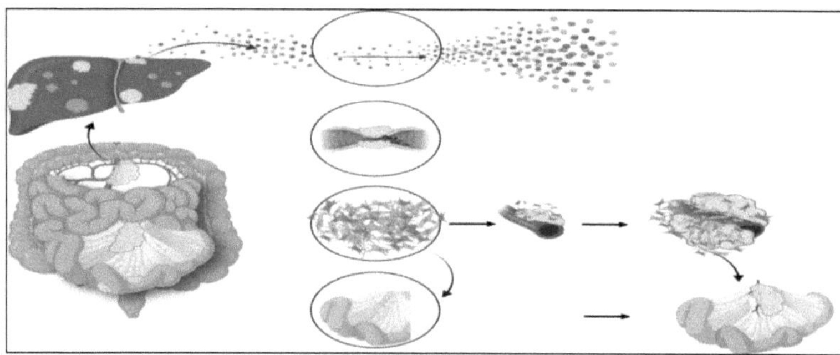

Figure 22: Secretion and formation of mesenteric fibrosis

meurs (75-77). Patients undergoing emergency surgery often have an incomplete initial resection, but may benefit from revision surgery to perform a radical resection including appropriate mesenteric lymph node curage (76,77). Primary NNEGs occur most frequently in the distal ileum, within 60-80 cm of the ileo-caecal valve, and less frequently in the proximal ileum or jejunum. Occasional caecal tumours with serotonin immunoreactivity are classified as NNEG (28). The primary tumor is usually a small, flat, fibrous submucosal lesion; they may also be polypoid (78).

Tumors can be difficult to detect surgically, often manifesting only as localized fibrosis or thickening of the intestinal wall, but can even in cases of minimal fibrosis cause intestinal obstruction (78). In one series, more than 30% of patients operated on had multiple submucosal tumour nodules in the wall of the small intestine, close to the primary tumour, which could represent local lymphatic dissemination (78,79). Rare cases have presented additional, larger polyps in the proximal intestine, possibly representing additional primary tumours (78). Mesenteric metastases occur with high frequency, irrespective of tumour size, and their microscopic spread has been almost invariably present (77,78). When developing close to the intestinal wall, metastases can easily be confused with primary tumours, and some primary tumours are confused with lymph node metastases (42,78). Mesenteric metastases are often larger than the primary tumour and may provoke a desmoplastic reaction with typically pronounced mesenteric fibrosis constituting the mesenteric complex (80).fibrosis may be due to the local effects of serotonin, growth factors and other substances released by NNEG metastases (81). Larger metastases and more extensive fibrosis cause contraction of the mesentery at the mesenteric root in the retroperitoneum, with a fibrous connection to the horizontal duodenum (42). These mesenteric tumors can extend upwards into the mesenteric root, and can sometimes grow into the duodenal wall or pancreas, or spread to the hepato duodenal ligament or para-aortic retroperitoneal spaces (80). These fibrous attachments can bend and wedge the intestines, causing subocclusion or OIA of the small intestine and, in advanced stages, sometimes duodenal obstruction (81).

With extensive mesenteric tumor growth and fibrosis, the mesenteric vessels may become enveloped and intestinal segments of variable length will appear reddish-blue due to incipient venous ischemia. The patient may present with diarrhea or functional obstruction and sometimes intestinal angina (80). A specific angiopathy, called vascular elastosis, with proliferation of elastic tissue in the adventitia and marked thickening of mesenteric vessel walls has been reported with advanced NNEG (82).

Cases presenting with tumors of the superior mesenteric root and occlusion of the superior mesenteric vein or artery may have large intestinal segments involved with pale blue cyanosis or sometimes absent arterial circulation. Rare patients with occlusion of a larger mesenteric venous branch may present with a condition similar to the WDHA syndrome seen in VIPOME, severe watery diarrhea, malnutrition and emaciation (83). If the tumour and fibrosis persist for longer, adhesions and intestinal strictures will create a conglomerate of intestinal loops sometimes attached to the abdominal wall, which is why some authors advocate resection of the primary tumour, even if asymptomatic in its early stages, or even in the presence of unresectable liver metastases (84,85).

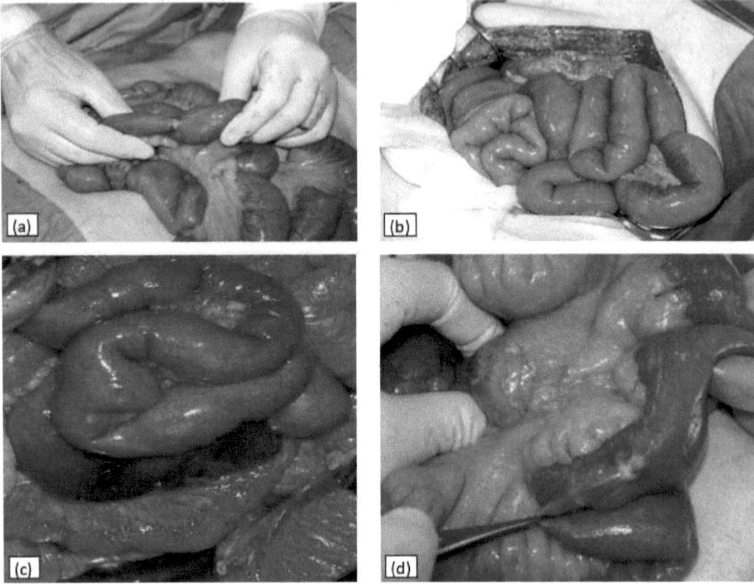

Figure 23: Local consequences of disease:(a) obstruction, (b)early ischemia, (c) advanced ischemia, (d) mesenteric complex.

1.6.4 Appendicular NETs:

They are usually revealed by an appendicular syndrome, undergo emergency surgery and are diagnosed by routine pathological examination. These tumors may be associated with lymph node metastases, but this risk is related to several pathological features (75). In patients with tumors <1 cm, healthy resection margins and no appendicular perforation, the risk is nil and no reoperation is necessary. Conversely, re-operation for right colectomy with lymph node dissection is indicated for patients with tumors >2 cm, or tumors comprising both endocrine and exocrine components. Between these two thresholds, reintervention for right colectomy or follow-up should be proposed according to age, general condition, grade and margins on the appendectomy specimen, and after discussion in the RCP (75).

1.6.5 Rectal NETs:

They are often diagnosed incidentally following colonoscopy with resection of a small, yellowish rectal polyp (<1 to 2 cm). Because of the submucosal origin of rectal NETs, endoscopic resection of incidental tumors is often not radical (R1). For tumors <1 cm, local endoscopic resection is curative provided that a radical resection (R0) is obtained, so no reoperation is necessary. For tumors > 2 cm, the risk of lymph node metastases is high, and reoperation for proctectomy with excision of the mesorectum (to obtain adequate lymph node curage and healthy margins) is indicated. Between these 2 thresholds, the choice between trans-anal reintervention and proctectomy with excision of the mesorectum must be determined according to age, location, lymph node staging (MRI and/or endoscopic ultrasound) and grade (75).

1.6.6 Pancreatic NNE (NNEP):

Their overall prognosis is good. However, their biological behavior is highly heterogeneous (functional or not) and their prognostic spectrum is equally broad, ranging from totally benign to very aggressive tumors. Overall, complete surgical resection is the only curative treatment that should be offered whenever possible, taking into consideration the low immediate risk and the low long-term functional impairment.

In practice, indications for resection must be adapted according to the clinical presentation (tumor discovered incidentally or symptomatically, sporadic or genetic predisposition), the presence or absence of a hormonal syndrome (functional or non-functional NNEP), the type of hormonal secretion (the most common being insulin and gastrin), histoprognostic factors (including tumour stage and grade) and the patient's general condition (age, comorbidities).

I.6.6.1 NNEP-Functional :

I.6.6.1.1 Insulinomas :

They are generally small in size (usually 1-2 cm), which frequently makes diagnosis difficult, and are benign in 95% of cases, with a very low risk of recurrence (5%) after resection. After appropriate clinical and biological diagnosis (fasting test demonstrating hypoglycemia and inappropriate serum insulin and C-peptide levels), the tumor must be localized by CT scan, MRI and or echo-endoscopy. Together, these three procedures can localize up to 95% of insulinomas (86). Exceptionally, other imaging procedures (GLP-1 scintigraphy or contrast-enhanced echo-endoscopy) are required. Approximately 5% of insulinomas are associated with multiple endocrine neoplasia type 1 and may be multiple or coexist with other non-functional NNEP (75). Surgical resection is almost always proposed because of the severity of symptoms, poor long-term efficacy and tolerance to medical treatment (diazoxide), and is often conservative because of the benignity of the disease (grade 1 is extremely common, and lymph node or liver metastases are exceptional) (87).Intraoperatively, tumour location can be determined more precisely with intraoperative ultrasound. Insulinomas located more than 1 to 2 mm from the Wirsung duct are suitable for enucleation, if possible laparoscopically, with a high risk of postoperative complications (pancreatic fistula) but no risk of long-term pancreatic insufficiency, as no parenchyma is resected(87- 90). Conversely, for anatomical reasons (relationship of the insulinoma to the Wirsung duct), around a third of patients require a regulated pancreatectomy (distal or cephalic), with a small but real mortality risk (1-3%) and a 20-30% risk of surgery-induced diabetes in the long term (87-90). The rate of patients definitively cured by surgery varies from 90% to 9% (75,87). In patients at high operative risk, ablative therapy (EUS-guided radiofrequency ablation) is an alternative to enucleation(91). EUS-guided ethanol ablation of insulinomas is another new treatment method also recommended for patients who are poor candidates for surgery or who refuse surgery (92). For insulinomas developed on MEN-1 multiple endocrine disease, multiple enucleations or distal pancreatectomy with cephalic enucleations may be proposed.

In summary, surgical treatment of insulinoma is primarily a technical problem, as prolonged medical treatment is generally not possible and the tumor disease has a benign behavior. Resection of insulinoma requires precise localization of the tumour pre- and intraoperatively, and must include preservation of the parenchyma as often as possible.

I.6.6.1.2 Gastrinomas :

Zollinger Ellison Syndrome (ZES), but also gastrointestinal bleeding from the upper digestive tract or perforated peptic ulcer as possible inaugural complications. The diagnosis can be evoked when symptoms are corrected by proton pump inhibitors, particularly when high doses are required, and confirmed by oeso-gastroduodenal fibroscopy, CT scan and somatostatin receptor scintigraphy (SRS). Although gastrinomas are almost always located in the duodeno-pancreatic zone, cross-sectional imaging frequently fails to localize gastrinomas and their extension, due to their small size (<1 cm), their duodenal site in 2/3 of cases, their multiplicity in 10-20% of cases (even sporadic), and the presence of lymph node metastases in 60% of cases. Because of these characteristics, echo-endoscopy and/or PET Ga 68 are often necessary (75,93,94). In addition, 20-25% of gastrinoma patients have NEM-1, which should be systematically investigated. Gastrinomas are predominantly malignant in behavior, although tumor progression is generally slow due to the high prevalence of grade 1 and low grade 2. Node invasion and the liver are the most frequent metastatic sites, suggesting that

MRI of the liver with diffusion-weighted sequences should be routinely performed (21,22). Once ZES has been diagnosed (or even strongly suspected), priority is given to PPI therapy to completely inhibit acid hypersecretion, using high doses if necessary. Surgery should be discussed once symptoms have disappeared and after a full work-up. The main aim of surgery is to prevent the development of liver metastases, which is the main prognostic factor (93).

In patients with sporadic gastrinoma, surgery is mainly indicated in patients without distant metastases, and should include tumour resection (by duodenotomy for duodenal localizations; or by enucleation or pancreatectomy for pancreatic localizations) (93) associated with systematic lymph node curage (95). Intraoperatively, routine pancreatic ultrasound and duodenotomy are useful for improving tumour detection and localization. Surgery seems capable of improving overall survival (compared with non-operated patients) (96), but definitive cure of gas- trine hypersecretion is more rarely observed, probably due to some small undiagnosed localizations left in place or persistent lymph node metastases (97). Surgery for metastatic gastrinoma, resecting primary tumours, lymph node and liver metastases, is rarely performed in highly selected patients. In MEN-1 patients, the multiplicity of secreting tumors means that local surgery (including lumpectomy + lymph node dissection) is not sufficient to effectively treat gastrin hypersecretion. For this purpose, cephalic duodenopancreatectomy (CPD) is more effective, but several authors are reluctant to perform it because of its high early and long-term morbidity (75). The risk of malignancy is only considered in patients with pancreatic NET > 2 cm, so surgery is generally only indicated in this subgroup of MEN-1 patients (75).

In summary, the surgical treatment of gastrinomas is primarily an oncological problem, as acid hypersecretion is easily controlled by PPI provided sufficient doses are used. Although the majority of gastrinomas are malignant (60% of lymph node metastases at diagnosis), tumor progression is generally slow. Radical surgery (in particular DPC) is rarely performed, and most authors prefer more limited surgery (lumpectomy + lymph node curage) to limit the risk of distant metastatic progression, with few postoperative complications and functional disorders.

I.6.6.1.3 Other functional pancreatic tumors :

This group mainly comprises VIPoma, glucagonoma and somatostati- noma, which are generally large and malignant (75).

In VIPoma patients, the priority is to treat the consequences of hypersecretion (diarrhea with hypokalemia), generally with somatostatin analogues. When resectable, these tumors generally require a regulated pancreatectomy with lymph node curage.

I.6.6.2Non-functional NNEP-NF :

The incidence of non-functional NNEP (NNEP-NF) has risen considerably over the past 20 years, from 1.7/100,000 in 1973-1977 to 4.3/100,000 in 2003-2007 (43). This increase is particularly marked for small NNEP-NF, whose incidence has risen by 700% in 20 years, due to the widespread diffusion of cross-sectional imaging, which detects more and more NNEP-NF (98), particularly small NNEP (≤2 cm). In recent series, incidentally diagnosed NNEP-NF account for up to 50% of patients operated on (96,99). Conversely, symptomatic NNEP-NF are revealed by symptoms of pain or compression, may be large, locally advanced or even metastatic (100,101). The histo-pronostic characteristics of NNEP-NF vary widely. They have been determined in surgical series, which mainly included patients with non-metastatic disease, with possible bias at least by limiting the number of G3 tumors. Histoprognostic characteristics are mainly related to tumor size. The 2 cm threshold is frequently used in the literature because :

• Represents the boundary between T1 and T2 tumors in the TNM classification proposed by UICC and ENETS;

• Clinically relevant because of its prognostic value (55,97,102).

• Close to the average diameter of resected NNEP-NF since half (30 to 65%) of NNEP-NF have a diameter ≤2 cm (55,96,99) .

According to these surgical series, it is possible to estimate the rate of lymph node metastases (as a predictive factor of tumor aggressiveness) close to 10% and the probability of a G2 / G3 grade at 15-20% for NNEP-NF ≤ 2 cm. However, this size, measured by macroscopic examination, may be smaller than that measured by imaging, probably due to the loss of arterial hyper vascularization after resection (103). Otherwise, 2 series showed that the absence of symptoms (incidental diagnosis) was associated with a higher chance of "benign behavior" and a better prognosis (55,96). Finally, in a multicenter study, the absence of ductal dilatation (biliary and/or pancreatic) was an independent factor associated with better recurrence-free survival (104).

I.6.6.2.1 Pancreatic surgery for NNEP-NF :

***Principles*: in the** past, non-functioning pancreatic neuroendocrine neoplasia was treated by "radical" pancreatectomy, combining parenchymal resection and lymph node curage: DPC or left pancreatectomy (PG) with or without splenectomy. Today, these procedures are performed with low mortality (2-5% after CPP, 1-3% after LP) in high-volume centers, but with early morbidity ranging from 30 to 50% (105-107). The long-term results of these procedures are characterized by a risk of de novo diabetes ranging from

10 to 20% after CPP and 10 to 35% after PG (108-110). The risk of de novo exocrine insufficiency requiring enzyme supplementation is higher after CPP than after PG (on average 60% versus 10% respectively) (111). Long-term pancreatic function has become an important issue in the decision to resect low-grade NNEP-NF, particularly in patients with incidentaloma. For this reason, *parenchyma-sparing pancreatectomies* (PSP), mainly enucleation (EN) and central pancreatectomy (CP), have been proposed to limit the loss of pancreatic function induced by surgery. Indeed, the risk of de novo diabetes is close to zero after EN and a maximum of 16% after CP, depending on the characteristics of the parenchyma and the extent of resection(106,110). After CP, the risk of exocrine insufficiency is less than 10%, which is significantly lower than that observed after DPC (111). The risk of exocrine insufficiency following EN is close to zero (89,110). However, PSP-sparing pancreatectomy has two limitations:

• Non-zero mortality after EN (89,110) or PC (106,112) due to surgical or medical complications;

• And early morbidity at least equivalent, if not superior, to "radical" pancreatectomy (89,106,110,112).

Indeed, average morbidity rates are around 60% and 45% in PC and EN, versus 50% and 30% in DPC and PG respectively (89,106,110,111). This morbidity is mainly due to pancreatic fistula, which occurs more frequently due to the proximity of the main pancreatic duct in EN(88,90) and the presence of two pancreatic cutting surfaces in CP (106,112).

What kind of operation for NNEP-NF?

I.6.6.2.2 Technical and functional aspects :

With regard to technical aspects, tumour location is important. Tumours located far (> 2 mm) from the main pancreatic duct are suitable for EN (88,90). Conversely, when the tumour is closer to, or even in contact with, the main pancreatic duct, the risk of ductal injury and postoperative fistula argues against EN and therefore for excision including parenchymal resection (DPC, PG or PC). The location in the pancreatic parenchyma (cephalic, central or distal) must be taken into account according to age and general condition. In particular, DPC and PC can be considered as in high-risk cases (elderly subjects or those with comorbidities) and, conversely, PG is better tolerated (107, 108). As regards long-term functional results, the better outcomes of sparing surgery (PSP) must be weighed against their higher early morbidity, particularly for CP whose alternative is PG. Thus, patients undergoing PSP should be fit enough to overcome the higher early morbidity of PSP(108). Moreover, young patients with a long life expectancy are more likely to benefit from PSP than elderly patients. Overall, the assessment of the balance between the benefits and risks of these operations for NNEP-NF, must take into account all these technical aspects but also age and general condition(108,113).For example, a small cephalic tumor (<2 cm) distant (> 2 mm) from the main pancreatic duct should ideally be enucleated to avoid the disadvantages of CPP, particularly in a high-risk patient. Conversely, a small tumor (<2 cm) in contact with the main pancreatic duct is not suitable for EN and can be resected by a short PG when localized in the tail, or by PC when isthmocorporeal.

1.6.6.2.3 Oncological aspects :

PSP does not include lymph node curage, but "picking" is possible. Indeed, in a retrospective study, lymph node curage was analyzed in 25% of PSP versus 97% of standard pancreatectomies (113). Thus, the oncological value of PSP is highly debated and these procedures are only justified for small (<2 cm), low-grade NNEP, which entails a low risk of lymph node metastasis and a high probability of expected cure. Histo-prognostic factors for NNEP ≤ 2 cm suggest that, for this subgroup of tumors, PSP is adequate and that, on the contrary, radical pancreatectomy is an "overtreatment" in around 90% of patients. It seems possible to propose PSP for every NNEP-NF ≤ 2 cm with a favorable presentation (no symptoms, no ductal dilatation, no detectable lymph node or liver metastases). Some authors have suggested a lower size threshold, between 1 cm and 1.7 cm (42-45). There is probably no single discriminating threshold in terms of size, and other criteria, including grade if available, are important. But the general idea is to avoid surgical over-treatment in asymptomatic patients, often over 60 years of age (114), and particularly in cases of cephalic localization.

1.6.6.2.4 Observation as an alternative to resection in small NNEP-NF

Because of the early risks and long-term consequences of pancreatectomies, the routine resection paradigm for every NNEP-NF has recently been reconsidered, particularly for small, asymptomatic tumors (incidentalomas). However, this approach requires accurate tumor characterization and a precise assessment of the benefit/risk ratio, taking into account tumor location and the patient's general condition.

I.6.7 Extended resection for locally advanced tumors :

Gastric or mainly pancreatic NNEP-NF NETs can be voluminous and may invade neighboring organs. In particular, they may envelop surrounding vessels or be responsible for endovascular extension leading to tumor thrombus. The resectability criteria for NNEP-NF are less restrictive than those for adenocarcinoma, so initial resection can frequently be attempted for these locally advanced tumours (96). Survival after resection is not impaired by microscopic involvement of the resection margins (101,115), and 5-year survival is around 50% after extensive radical resection of locally advanced NNEP (96). The role of neoadjuvant therapy, using systemic chemotherapy or PRRT radionuclide therapy (85), is still being evaluated.

I.6.8 Surgery of NNE GEP with liver metastases:

Surgery was also considered a "gold standard" to be offered whenever possible to patients with metastatic NNE (75). This approach was justified by the results of large single-center retrospective studies (84) or large multicenter databases (116), which reported better survival after resection of the primary tumor or liver metastases if possible, or both. When no major hepatectomy is required, resection of liver metastases can be performed at the same stage as resection of the primary tumour, if not at a second stage (117). Hepatic surgery can be facilitated by the use of ablative techniques (radiofrequency ablation, microwaves) for deep lesions <3 cm (118). This approach can be performed with a mortality of less than 5%, an overall survival of 80% at 5 years, but a 50% risk of hepatic recurrence due to unrecognized microscopic involvement at the time of surgery. To limit the risk of recurrence, preoperative evaluation of hepatic and extra-hepatic extension should use MRI with diffusion-weighted sequences(119)and probably Pet Ga 68 (94). It is also important to limit indications for hepatectomy to well-differentiated, low-grade tumours (G1 and low G2). The role of neoadjuvant treatment with systemic chemotherapy is currently being evaluated (120). When liver disease is unresectable, some authors have suggested resecting the primary to improve survival (84,85), avoid long-term complications related to the primary and then concentrate on treating the hepatic localization. This approach is highly controversial, as no prospective comparative studies are available (121). However, it is frequently used for small bowel primitives, which can be complicated by OIA in up to 25% of cases, or more rarely for distal pancreatic primitives (121). For cephalic pancreatic primitives, performing CPP usually precludes simultaneous extensive liver resection and also increases the septic complications of any subsequent liver therapy (resection, ablation or embolization) due to bacterial contamination of the biliary tree above the hepaticojejunal anastomosis (122). Exceptionally, diffuse bi-lobar liver metastases of NNE GEP can be treated by total hepatectomy and liver transplantation. The most favourable long-term results are obtained in young patients with a previously resected low-grade primary, and a limited tumour burden resulting in moderate hepatomegaly (123).

I.7 The multidisciplinary approach to the management of NNED :

Optimal management of neuroendocrine neoplasia (NEN) requires a multidisciplinary approach, involving specialists from diverse fields such as surgery, medical oncology, radiology, pathology and nuclear medicine. The importance of multidisciplinary approaches in the management of NNE D, with essential contributions from each disc ipline is the only guarantee of quality management.

1.7.1 The Role of Surgery:

Surgery remains the treatment of choice for many NNEDs, particularly for localized and functional tumors. Surgical procedures, such as tumor resection, lymphadenectomy, and liver cytoreduction surgery, aim to remove primary tumors and metastases, where appropriate (124). Minimally invasive surgical approaches, such as laparoscopy and robotics, have also been developed to reduce postoperative morbidity (125).

1.7.2 The Role of Medical Oncology :

Medical treatments, such as chemotherapy, targeted therapy and radionuclide therapy, are the oncological armamentarium used in the management of NNEDs. Medical oncologists are responsible for managing these treatments, taking into account the histological nature of NNEDs, their grade of differentiation, their functionality, and the presence of metastases (17). In addition, new targeted therapies, such as angiogenesis and pathway inhibition, have shown promising results in recent clinical trials (126).

1.7.3 The Role of Pathology:

Accurate pathological evaluation is crucial for the diagnosis and classification of NNE. Pathologists determine the grade of differentiation, assess cell proliferation, and identify speci- fic immunohistochemical markers. Accurate histological classification is essential to guide therapeutic decisions (127).

I.7.4 The Role of Radiology and Nuclear Medicine:

Medical imaging plays a key role in the diagnosis, staging, follow-up and assessment of response to treatment of NNED. CT, MRI, somatostatin scintigraphy, and somatostatin positron emission tomography (PET) are imaging modalities frequently used to visualize lesions and assess their extension (128). Moreover, in the age of theranos- tics, nuclear medicine offers innovative therapeutic options, such as metabolic radiotherapy based on PRRT radionuclides like 177 Lu- DOTATATE (129-131).

Bibliography

1. Lubarsch O. Ueber den primaren Krebs des Ileum nebst Bemerkungen über das gleichzeitige Vor- kommen von Krebs und Tuberculose. Archiv f pathol Anat. Feb 1888;111(2):280-317.

2. Drozdov I, Modlin IM, Kidd M, Goloubinov VV. Nikolai Konstantinovich Kulchitsky (1856-1925). J Med Biogr. Feb 2009;17(1):47-54.

3. JP SAINT ANDRÉ. Anatomie pathologique des tumeurs neuro-endocrines. e-mémoires de l'Académie Nationale de Chirurgie; 2003.

4. Arthur N'Golet. Endocrine cells of the gastric mucosa: a review of the literature [Internet]. 2013. Available from: https://dumas.ccsd.cnrs.fr/dumas-00833203

5. Moertel CG, Sauer WG, Dockerty MB, Baggenstoss AH. Life history of the carcinoid tumor of the small intestine. Cancer. 1961;14:901-12.

6. Moertel CG. Karnofsky memorial lecture. An odyssey in the land of small tumors. JCO. Oct 1987;5(10):1502-22.

7. Howe JR. Carcinoid Tumors: Past, Present, and Future. Indian J Surg Oncol. June 2020;11(2):182-7.

8. Bussolati G. C and APUD Cells and Endocrine Tumours. Pearse's Laboratory in the Years 1965-1969: A Personal Recollection. Endocr Pathol. June 2014;25(2):133-40.

9. De Mestier L, Lepage C, Baudin E, Coriat R, Courbon F, Couvelard A, et al. Digestive Neuroendocrine Neoplasms (NEN): French Intergroup clinical practice guidelines for diagnosis, treatment and followup (SNFGE, GTE, RENATEN, TENPATH, FFCD, GERCOR, UNICANCER, SFCD, SFED, SFRO, SFR). Digestive and Liver Disease. May 2020;52(5):473-92.

10. Hautefeuille vincent. Clinical characteristics and pre-therapeutic assessment of digestive neuroendocrine neoplasms. 2020;

11. Parikh A, Thevenin C. Physiology, Gastrointestinal Hormonal Control. In: StatPearls [Internet]. Treasure Island (FL): StatPearls Publishing; 2024 [cited 2024 Feb 10]. Available from: http://www.ncbi.nlm.nih.gov/books/NBK537284/

12. Fothergill LJ, Furness JB. Diversity of enteroendocrine cells investigated at cellular and subcellular levels: the need for a new classification scheme. Histochem Cell Biol. Dec 2018;150(6):693-702.

13. Latorre R, Sternini C, De Giorgio R, Greenwood-Van Meerveld B. Enteroendocrine cells: a review of their role in brain-gut communication. Neurogastroenterology Motil. May 2016;28(5):620-30.

14. Seino Y, Fukushima M, Yabe D. GIP and GLP-1, the two incretin hormones: Similarities and differences. J Diabetes Investig. 22 Apr 2010;1(1-2):8-23.

15. Martini F, Timmons MJ, Tallitsch RB. Human anatomy. 7th ed. Boston: Pearson Benjamin Cummings; 2012. 870 p.

16. Modlin IM, Oberg K, Chung DC, Jensen RT, De Herder WW, Thakker RV, et al. Gastroenteropancreatic neuroendocrine tumours. The Lancet Oncology. Jan 2008;9(1):61-72.

17. Oberg K, Knigge U, Kwekkeboom D, Perren A. Neuroendocrine gastro-entero-pancreatic tumors: ESMO Clinical Practice Guidelines for diagnosis, treatment and follow-up. Annals of Oncology. oct 2012;23:vii124-30.

18. Rindi G, Klimstra DS, Abedi-Ardekani B, Asa SL, Bosman FT, Brambilla E, et al. A common classification framework for neuroendocrine neoplasms: an International Agency for Research on Cancer (IARC) and World Health Organization (WHO) expert consensus proposal. Modern Pathology. dec 2018;31(12):1770-86.

19. Philippe Ruszniewski. Pancreatic neuroendocrine tumors. POST'U (2019). 2020;

20. Rindi G, Mete O, Uccella S, Basturk O, La Rosa S, Brosens LAA, et al. Overview of the 2022 WHO Classification of Neuroendocrine Neoplasms. Endocr Pathol. March 2022;33(1):115-54.

21. Van Velthuysen MF, Couvelard A, Rindi G, Fazio N, Horsch D, Nieveen Van Dijkum EJ, et al. ENETS standardized (synoptic) reporting for neuroendocrine tumour pathology. J Neuroendocrinology. March 2022;34(3):e13100.

22. Mete O. Special Issue On the 2022 WHO Classification of Endocrine and Neuroendocrine Tumors: a New Primer for Endocrine Pathology Practice. Endocr Pathol. March 2022;33(1):1-2.

23. Juhlin CC, Zedenius J, Hoog A. Metastatic Neuroendocrine Neoplasms of Unknown Primary: Clues from Pathology Workup. Cancers. 28 Apr 2022;14(9):2210.

24. zammouchi Asma. histopronostic factors in digestive neuroendocrine tumors. thesis. université Saad Dahleb Blida; 2023.

25. Dasari A, Shen C, Halperin D, Zhao B, Zhou S, Xu Y, et al. Trends in the Incidence, Prevalence, and Survival Outcomes in Patients With Neuroendocrine Tumors in the United States. JAMA Oncol. 1 Oct 2017;3(10):1335.

26. Nagtegaal ID, Odze RD, Klimstra D, Paradis V, Rugge M, Schirmacher P, et al. The 2019 WHO classification of tumours of the digestive system. Histopathology. january 2020;76(2):182-8.

27. Couvelard A, Scoazec JY. Predisposition syndromes for gastroenteropancreatic and thoracic neuroendocrine tumors. Annales de Pathologie. Apr 2020;40(2):120-33.

28. Modlin IM, Oberg K, Chung DC, Jensen RT, De Herder WW, Thakker RV, et al. Gastroenteropancreatic neuroendocrine tumours. The Lancet Oncology. Jan 2008;9(1):61-72.

29. Hauso O, Gustafsson BI, Kidd M, Waldum HL, Drozdov I, Chan AKC, et al. Neuroendocrine

tumor epidemiology: Contrasting Norway and North America. Cancer. 15 Nov 2008;113(10):2655-64.

30. Yao JC, Hassan M, Phan A, Dagohoy C, Leary C, Mares JE, et al. One Hundred Years After "Carcinoid": Epidemiology of and Prognostic Factors for Neuroendocrine Tumors in 35,825 Cases in the United States. JCO. June 20, 2008;26(18):3063-72.

31. Das S, Dasari A. Epidemiology, Incidence, and Prevalence of Neuroendocrine Neoplasms: Are There Global Differences? Curr Oncol Rep. Apr 2021;23(4):43.

32. Fraenkel M, Kim MK, Faggiano A, Valk GD. Epidemiology of gastroenteropancreatic neuroendocrine tumours. Best Practice & Research Clinical Gastroenterology. dec 2012;26(6):691-703.

33. Hemminki K, Li X. Incidence trends and risk factors of carcinoid tumors: A nationwide epidemiologic study from Sweden. Cancer. 15 Oct 2001;92(8):2204-10.

34. Tsai HJ, Wu CC, Tsai CR, Lin SF, Chen LT, Chang JS. The Epidemiology of Neuroendocrine Tumors in Taiwan: A Nation-Wide Cancer Registry-Based Study. Gorlova OY, editor. PLoS ONE. Apr 22, 2013;8(4):e62487.

35. McCullough ML, Jacobs EJ, Shah R, Campbell PT, Wang Y, Hartman TJ, et al. Meat consumption and pancreatic cancer risk among men and women in the Cancer Prevention Study-II Nutrition Cohort. Cancer Causes Control. Jan 2018;29(1):125-33.

36. Field RW, Withers BL. Occupational and environmental causes of lung cancer. Clin Chest Med. Dec 2012;33(4):681-703.

37. Xu Z, Wang L, Dai S, Chen M, Li F, Sun J, et al. Epidemiologic Trends of and Factors Associated With Overall Survival for Patients With Gastroenteropancreatic Neuroendocrine Tumors in the United States. JAMA Netw Open. 23 Sep 2021;4(9):e2124750.

38. JNETS Project Study Group, Masui T, Ito T, Komoto I, Uemoto S. Recent epidemiology of patients with gastro-entero-pancreatic neuroendocrine neoplasms (GEP-NEN) in Japan: a population-based study. BMC Cancer. Dec 2020;20(1):1104.

39. Grozinsky-Glasberg S, Davar J, Hofland J, Dobson R, Prasad V, Pascher A, et al. European Neuroendocrine Tumor Society (ENETS) 2022 Guidance Paper for Carcinoid Syndrome and Carcinoid Heart Disease. J Neuroendocrinology. Jul 2022;34(7):e13146.

40. Zhang C, Huang Y, Long J, Yao X, Wang J, Zang S, et al. Serum chromogranin A for the diagnosis of gastroenteropancreatic neuroendocrine neoplasms and its association with tumour expression. Oncol Lett [Internet]. 5 Dec 2018 [cited 24 Sep 2023]; Available from: http://www.spandidos- publications.com/10.3892/ol.2018.9795

41. Frilling A, Âkerstrõm G, Falconi M, Pavel M, Ramos J, Kidd M, et al. Neuroendocrine tumor disease: an evolving landscape. Endocrine-Related Cancer. oct 2012;19(5):R163-85.

42. Âkerstrõm G, Hellman P, Hessman O. Midgut carcinoid tumours: surgical treatment and prognosis. Best Practice & Research Clinical Gastroenterology. Oct 2005;19(5):717-28.

43. Lawrence B, Gustafsson BI, Chan A, Svejda B, Kidd M, Modlin IM. The Epidemiology of Gastroentero- pancreatic Neuroendocrine Tumors. Endocrinology and Metabolism Clinics of North America. March 2011;40(1):1-18.

44. Granberg D, Wilander E, Stridsberg M, Granerus G, Skogseid B, Oberg K. Clinical symptoms, hormone profiles, treatment, and prognosis in patients with gastric carcinoids. Gut. 1998;43:223-8.

45. Jensen EH, Kvols L, McLoughlin JM, Lewis JM, Alvarado MD, Yeatman T, et al. Biomarkers Predict Outcomes Following Cytoreductive Surgery for Hepatic Metastases from Functional Carcinoid Tumors. Ann Surg Oncol. Feb 2007;14(2):780-5.

46. Pavel M, O''Toole D, Costa F, Capdevila J, Gross D, Kianmanesh R, et al. ENETS Consensus Guidelines Update for the Management of Distant Metastatic Disease of Intestinal, Pancreatic, Bronchial Neuroendocrine Neoplasms (NEN) and NEN of Unknown Primary Site. Neuroendocrinology. 2016;103(2):172-85.

47. Banck MS, Kanwar R, Kulkarni AA, Boora GK, Metge F, Kipp BR, et al. The genomic landscape of small intestine neuroendocrine tumors. J Clin Invest. June 3, 2013;123(6):2502-8.

48. Ruf J, Heuck F, Schiefer J, Denecke T, Elgeti F, Pascher A, et al. Impact of Multiphase^{68} Ga-DOTATOC- PET/CT on Therapy Management in Patients with Neuroendocrine Tumors. Neuroendocrinology. 2010;91(1):101-9.

49. Sundin A. Radiological and nuclear medicine imaging of gastroenteropancreatic neuroendocrine tumours. Best Practice & Research Clinical Gastroenterology. dec 2012;26(6):803-18.

50. Pirasteh A, Lovrec P, Bodei L. Imaging of neuroendocrine tumors: A pictorial review of the clinical value of different imaging modalities. Rev Endocr Metab Disord. Sept 2021;22(3):539-52.

51. Zhao Q, Dong A, He T, Zuo C. Somatostatin Receptor PET Imaging in Diffuse Pancreatic Neuroendocrine Tumor. Clin Nucl Med. May 2023;48(5):453-6.

52. Prosperi D, Gentiloni Silveri G, Panzuto F, Faggiano A, Russo V, Caruso D, et al. Nuclear Medicine and Radiological Imaging of Pancreatic Neuroendocrine Neoplasms: A Multidisciplinary Update. JCM. 18 Nov 2022;11(22):6836.

53. Danti G, Flammia F, Matteuzzi B, Cozzi D, Berti V, Grazzini G, et al. Gastrointestinal neuroendocrine neoplasms (GI-NENs): hot topics in morphological, functional, and prognostic imaging. Radiol med. Dec 2021;126(12):1497-507.

54. Duan H, Iagaru A. Neuroendocrine Tumor Diagnosis. PET Clinics. Apr 2023;18(2):259-66.

55. Bettini R, Partelli S, Boninsegna L, Capelli P, Crippa S, Pederzoli P, et al. Tumor size correlates with malignancy in nonfunctioning pancreatic endocrine tumor. Surgery. Jul 2011;150(1):75-82.

56. Rindi G, Kloppel G, Alhman H, Caplin M, Couvelard A, De Herder WW, et al. TNM staging of foregut (neuro)endocrine tumors: a consensus proposal including a grading system.

Virchows Arch. Oct 2006;449(4):395-401.

57. World Health Organization, International Agency for Research on Cancer, editors. WHO classification of tumours of endocrine organs. 4th ed. Lyon: International agency for research on cancer; 2017. (World health organization classification of tumours).

58. Busico A, Maisonneuve P, Prinzi N, Pusceddu S, Centonze G, Garzone G, et al. Gastroenteropancreatic High-Grade Neuroendocrine Neoplasms: Histology and Molecular Analysis, Two Sides of the Same Coin. Neuroendocrinology. 2020;110(7-8):616-29.

59. Figueiredo MN, Maggiori L, Gaujoux S, Couvelard A, Guedj N, Ruszniewski P, et al. Surgery for smallbowel neuroendocrine tumors: Is there any benefit of the laparoscopic approach? Surg Endosc. May 2014;28(5):1720-6.

60. de Mestier. de Mestier L, Walter T, Hadoux S, Cros J, Deguelte S, Gaujoux S, Hautefeuille V, Imperiale A, Laboureau S, Perrier M, Ronot M, Lepage C, Goichot B, Bouché O, Cadiot G. "Neoplasies Neuroendocrines Digestives". Thésaurus National de Cancérologie Digestive, November 2023, [http://www.tncd.org]. 2023.

61. Eriksson B, Kloppel G, Krenning E, Ahlman H, Plockinger U, Wiedenmann B, et al. Consensus Guidelines for the Management of Patients with Digestive Neuroendocrine Tumors - Well-Differentiated Jejunal-Ileal Tumor/Carcinoma. Neuroendocrinology. 2008;87(1):8-19.

62. Elias D, Debaere T, Roche A, Bonvallot S, Lasser P. Preoperative selective portal vein embolizations are an effective means of extending the indications of major hepatectomy in the normal and injured liver. Hepatogastroenterology. 1998;45(19):170-7.

63. Adam R, Laurent A, Azoulay D, Castaing D, Bismuth H. Two-Stage Hepatectomy: A Planned Strategy to Treat Irresectable Liver Tumors: Annals of Surgery. Dec 2000;232(6):777-85.

64. Gough I. **Endocrine Surgery. A Companion to Specialist Surgical Practice**. ANZ Journal of Surgery. May 2002;72(5):381-381.

65. Sorbye H, Welin S, Langer SW, Vestermark LW, Holt N, Osterlund P, et al. Predictive and prognostic factors for treatment and survival in 305 patients with advanced gastrointestinal neuroendocrine carcinoma (WHO G3): The NORDIC NEC study. Annals of Oncology. Jan 2013;24(1):152-60.

66. Ilett E, Langer S, Olsen I, Federspiel B, Kjær A, Knigge U. Neuroendocrine Carcinomas of the Gas- troenteropancreatic System: A Comprehensive Review. Diagnostics. 8 Apr 2015;5(2):119-76.

67. Lloyd RV, Osamura RY, Kloppel G, Rosai J. WHO Classification of Tumours of Endocrine Organs WHO Classification of Tumours, 4th Edition, Volume 10. In: WHO classification of tumours of endocrine organs 4th ed World Health Organization, International Agency for Research on Cancer, publishers.

68. Rindi G, Luinetti O, Cornaggia M, Capella C, Solcia E. Three subtypes of gastric argyrophil carcinoid and the gastric neuroendocrine carcinoma: A clinicopathologic study. Gastroenterology. Apr 1993;104(4):994-1006.

69. O'Toole D, Delle Fave G, Jensen RT. Gastric and duodenal neuroendocrine tumours. Best Practice & Research Clinical Gastroenterology. dec 2012;26(6):719-35.

70. Ruszniewski P, Delle Fave G, Cadiot G, Komminoth P, Chung D, Kos-Kudla B, et al. Well-Differentiated Gastric Tumors/Carcinomas. Neuroendocrinology. 2006;84(3):158-64.

71. Borch K, Ahrén B, Ahlman H, Falkmer S, Granérus G, Grimelius L. Gastric Carcinoids: Biologic Behavior and Prognosis After Differentiated Treatment in Relation to Type. Annals of Surgery. July 2005;242(1):64-73.

72. Sok C, Ajay PS, Tsagkalidis V, Kooby DA, Shah MM. Management of Gastric Neuroendocrine Tumors: A Review. Ann Surg Oncol. March 2024;31(3):1509-18.

73. Ahmed M. Gastrointestinal neuroendocrine tumors in 2020. WJGO. August 15, 2020;12(8):791-807.

74. Berge T, Linell F. Carcinoid tumours. Frequency in a defined population during a 12-year period. Acta Pathol Microbiol Scand A. July 1976;84(4):322-30.

75. O'Toole D, Kianmanesh R, Caplin M. ENETS 2016 Consensus Guidelines for the Management of Patients with Digestive Neuroendocrine Tumors: An Update. Neuroendocrinology. 2016;103(2):117-8.

76. Landry CS, Lin HY, Phan A, Charnsangavej C, Abdalla EK, Aloia T, et al. Resection of At-Risk Mesenteric Lymph Nodes Is Associated with Improved Survival in Patients with Small Bowel Neuroendocrine Tumors. World J Surg. Jul 2013;37(7):1695-700.

77. Motz BM, Lorimer PD, Boselli D, Hill JS, Salo JC. Optimal Lymphadenectomy in Small Bowel Neuroendocrine Tumors: Analysis of the NCDB. J Gastrointest Surg. jan 2018;22(1):117-23.

78. Makridis C, Oberg K, Juhlin C, Rastad J, Johansson H, Lorelius LE, et al. Surgical treatment of mid-gut carcinoid tumors. World j surg. May 1990;14(3):377-83.

79. Guo Z, Li Q, Wilander E, Ponton J. Clonality analysis of multifocal carcinoid tumours of the small intestine by X-chromosome inactivation analysis. J Pathol. Jan 2000;190(1):76-9.

80. Ohrvall U, Eriksson B, Juhlin C, Karacagil S, Rastad J, Hellman P, et al. Method for Dissection of Mesenteric Metastases in Mid-gut Carcinoid Tumors. World j surg. nov 2000;24(11):1402-8.

81. Kidd M, Modlin IM. Small intestinal neuroendocrine cell pathobiology: 'carcinoid' tumors. Current Opinion in Oncology. Jan 2011;23(1):45-52.

82. Harvey JN, Denyer ME, DaCosta P. Intestinal infarction caused by carcinoid associated elastic vascular sclerosis: early presentation of a small ileal carcinoid tumour. Gut. May 1, 1989;30(5):691-4.

83. Vinik AI, McLeod MK, Fig LM, Shapiro B, Lloyd RV, Cho K. Clinical features, diagnosis, and localization of carcinoid tumors and their management. Gastroenterol Clin North Am. 1989.

84. Hüttner FJ, Schneider L, Tarantino I, Warschkow R, Schmied BM, Hackert T, et al. Palliative

resection of the primary tumor in 442 metastasized neuroendocrine tumors of the pancreas: a populationbased, propensity score-matched survival analysis. Langenbecks Arch Surg. August 2015;400(6):715-23.

85. Partelli S, Bertani E, Bartolomei M, Perali C, Muffatti F, Grana CM, et al. Peptide receptor radionuclide therapy as neoadjuvant therapy for resectable or potentially resectable pancreatic neuroendocrine neoplasms. Surgery. Apr 2018;163(4):761-7.

86. Gouya H, Vignaux O, Augui J, Dousset B, Palazzo L, Louvel A, et al. CT, Endoscopic Sonography, and a Combined Protocol for Preoperative Evaluation of Pancreatic Insulinomas. American Journal of Roentgenology. Oct 2003;181(4):987-92.

87. Nikfarjam M, Warshaw AL, Axelrod L, Deshpande V, Thayer SP, Ferrone CR, et al. Improved Contemporary Surgical Management of Insulinomas: A 25-year Experience at the Massachusetts General Hospital. Annals of Surgery. Jan 2008;247(1):165-72.

88. Brient C, Regenet N, Sulpice L, Brunaud L, Mucci-Hennekine S, Carrère N, et al. Risk Factors for Postoperative Pancreatic Fistulization Subsequent to Enucleation. J Gastrointest Surg. oct 2012;16(10):1883-7.

89. Faitot F, Gaujoux S, Barbier L, Novaes M, Dokmak S, Aussilhou B, et al. Reappraisal of pancreatic enucleations: A single-center experience of 126 procedures. Surgery. jul 2015;158(1):201-10.

90. Heeger K, Falconi M, Partelli S, Waldmann J, Crippa S, Fendrich V, et al. Increased rate of clinically relevant pancreatic fistula after deep enucleation of small pancreatic tumors. Langenbecks Arch Surg. March 2014;399(3):315-21.

91. Barthet M, Giovannini M, Lesavre N, Boustiere C, Napoleon B, Koch S, et al. Endoscopic ultrasound- guided radiofrequency ablation for pancreatic neuroendocrine tumors and pancreatic cystic neoplasms: a prospective multicenter study. Endoscopy. Sept 2019;51(09):836-42.

92. Dqbkowski K, Gajewska P, Walter K, Londzin-Olesik M, Biatek A, Andrysiak-Mammos E, et al. Successful EUS-guided ethanol ablation of insulinoma, four-year follow-up. Case report and literature review. Endokrynologia Polska. August 10, 2017;68(4):472-9.

93. Norton JA, Fraker DL, Alexander HR, Gibril F, Liewehr DJ, Venzon DJ, et al. Surgery Increases Survival in Patients With Gastrinoma. Annals of Surgery. Sept 2006;244(3):410-9.

94. Partelli S, Rinzivillo M, Maurizi A, Panzuto F, Salgarello M, Polenta V, et al. The Role of Combined^{68} Ga-DOTANOC and^{18} FDG PET/CT in the Management of Patients with Pancreatic Neuroendocrine Tumors. Neuroendocrinology. 2014;100(4):293-9.

95. Bartsch DK, Waldmann J, Fendrich V, Boninsegna L, Lopez CL, Partelli S, et al. Impact of lympha- denectomy on survival after surgery for sporadic gastrinoma. British Journal of Surgery. August 2, 2012;99(9):1234-40.

96. Birnbaum DJ, Gaujoux S, Cherif R, Dokmak S, Fuks D, Couvelard A, et al. Sporadic nonfunctioning pancreatic neuroendocrine tumors: Prognostic significance of incidental diagnosis. Surgery. jan 2014;155(1):13-21.

97. Scarpa A, Mantovani W, Capelli P, Beghelli S, Boninsegna L, Bettini R, et al. Pancreatic endocrine tumors: improved TNM staging and histopathological grading permit a clinically efficient prognostic stratification of patients. Modern Pathology. June 2010;23(6):824-33.

98. Kuo EJ, Salem RR. Population-Level Analysis of Pancreatic Neuroendocrine Tumors 2 cm or Less in Size. Ann Surg Oncol. sept 2013;20(9):2815-21.

99. Haynes AB. Implications of Incidentally Discovered, Nonfunctioning Pancreatic Endocrine Tumors: Short-term and Long-term Patient Outcomes. Arch Surg. May 1, 2011;146(5):534.

100. Bilimoria KY, Talamonti MS, Tomlinson JS, Stewart AK, Winchester DP, Ko CY, et al. Prognostic Score Predicting Survival After Resection of Pancreatic Neuroendocrine Tumors: Analysis of 3851 Patients. Annals of Surgery. March 2008;247(3):490-500.

101. Fischer L, Bergmann F, Schimmack S, Hinz U, Prieβ S, Müller-Stich BP, et al. Outcome of surgery for pancreatic neuroendocrine neoplasms. British Journal of Surgery. 8 Sep 2014;101(11):1405-12.

102. Ellison TA, Wolfgang CL, Shi C, Cameron JL, Murakami P, Mun LJ, et al. A Single Institution's 26Year Experience With Nonfunctional Pancreatic Neuroendocrine Tumors: A Validation of Current Staging Systems and a New Prognostic Nomogram. Annals of Surgery. feb 2014;259(2):204-12.

103. Partelli S, Gaujoux S, Boninsegna L, Cherif R, Crippa S, Couvelard A, et al. Pattern and Clinical Predictors of Lymph Node Involvement in Nonfunctioning Pancreatic Neuroendocrine Tumors (NF- PanNETs). JAMA Surg. Oct 1, 2013;148(10):932.

104. Sallinen VJ, Le Large TYS, Tieftrunk E, Galeev S, Kovalenko Z, Haugvik SP, et al. Prognosis of sporadic resected small (≤2 cm) nonfunctional pancreatic neuroendocrine tumors - a multi-institutional study. HPB. march 2018;20(3):251-9.

105. Farges O, Bendersky N, Truant S, Delpero JR, Pruvot FR, Sauvanet A. The Theory and Practice of Pancreatic Surgery in France. Annals of Surgery. nov 2017;266(5):797-804.

106. Iacono C, Verlato G, Ruzzenente A, Campagnaro T, Bacchelli C, Valdegamberi A, et al. Systematic review of central pancreatectomy and meta-analysis of central *versus* distal pancreatectomy. British Journal of Surgery. 2013 May 3;100(7):873-85.

107. Meguid RA, Ahuja N, Chang DC. What Constitutes a "High-Volume" Hospital for Pancreatic Resection? Journal of the American College of Surgeons. Apr 2008;206(4):622e1-9.

108. Cherif R, Gaujoux S, Couvelard A, Dokmak S, Vuillerme MP, Ruszniewski P, et al. ParenchymaSparing Resections for Pancreatic Neuroendocrine Tumors. J Gastrointest Surg. nov 2012;16(11):2045-55.

109. Falconi M, Mantovani W, Crippa S, Mascetta G, Salvia R, Pederzoli P. Pancreatic insufficiency after different resections for benign tumours. British Journal of Surgery. 28 Dec 2007;95(1):85-91.

110. Hüttner FJ, Koessler-Ebs J, Hackert T, Ulrich A, Büchler MW, Diener MK. Meta-analysis of surgical outcome after enucleation *versus* standard resection for pancreatic neoplasms. British Journal of Surgery. 14 Jul 2015;102(9):1026-36.

111. Sabater L, Ausania F, Bakker OJ, Boadas J, Domínguez-Muñoz JE, Falconi M, et al. Evidence-based Guidelines for the Management of Exocrine Pancreatic Insufficiency After Pancreatic Surgery. Annals of Surgery. dec 2016;264(6):949-58.

112. Goudard Y, Gaujoux S, Dokmak S, Cros J, Couvelard A, Palazzo M, et al. Reappraisal of Central Pancreatectomy: A 12-Year Single-Center Experience. JAMA Surg. Apr 1, 2014;149(4):356.

113. Toste PA, Kadera BE, Tatishchev SF, Dawson DW, Clerkin BM, Muthusamy R, et al. Nonfunctional Pancreatic Neuroendocrine Tumors <2 cm on Preoperative Imaging are Associated with a Low Incidence of Nodal Metastasis and an Excellent Overall Survival. J Gastrointest Surg. dec 2013;17(12):2105-13.

114. Halfdanarson TR, Rabe KG, Rubin J, Petersen GM. Pancreatic neuroendocrine tumors (PNETs): incidence, prognosis and recent trend toward improved survival. Annals of Oncology. Oct 2008;19(10):1727-33.

115. Pomianowska E, Gladhaug IP, Grzyb K, R0sok BI, Edwin B, Bergestuen DS, et al. Survival following resection of pancreatic endocrine tumors: importance of R-status and the WHO and TNM classification systems. Scandinavian Journal of Gastroenterology. August 2010;45(7-8):971-9.

116. Franko J, Feng W, Yip L, Genovese E, Moser AJ. Non-functional Neuroendocrine Carcinoma of the Pancreas: Incidence, Tumor Biology, and Outcomes in 2,158 Patients. J Gastrointest Surg. March 2010;14(3):541-8.

117. Kianmanesh R, Sauvanet A, Hentic O, Couvelard A, Lévy P, Vilgrain V, et al. Two-step Surgery for Synchronous Bilobar Liver Metastases From Digestive Endocrine Tumors: A Safe Approach for Radical Resection. Annals of Surgery. Apr 2008;247(4):659-65.

118. Elias D, Goéré D, Leroux G, Dromain C, Leboulleux S, De Baere Th, et al. Combined liver surgery and RFA for patients with gastroenteropancreatic endocrine tumors presenting with more than 15 metastases to the liver. European Journal of Surgical Oncology (EJSO). Oct 2009;35(10):1092-7.

119. d'Assignies G, Couvelard A, Bahrami S, Vullierme MP, Hammel P, Hentic O, et al. Pancreatic Endocrine Tumors: Tumor Blood Flow Assessed with Perfusion CT Reflects Angiogenesis and Correlates with Prognostic Factors[1] . Radiology. Feb 2009;250(2):407-16.

120. Cloyd JM, Omichi K, Mizuno T, Kawaguchi Y, Tzeng CWD, Conrad C, et al. Preoperative Fluorouracil, Doxorubicin, and Streptozocin for the Treatment of Pancreatic Neuroendocrine Liver Metastases. Ann Surg Oncol. June 2018;25(6):1709-15.

121. Partelli S, Cirocchi R, Rancoita PMV, Muffatti F, Andreasi V, Crippa S, et al. A Systematic review and meta-analysis on the role of palliative primary resection for pancreatic neuroendocrine neoplasm with liver metastases. HPB. March 2018;20(3):197-203.

122. De Jong MC, Farnell MB, Sclabas G, Cunningham SC, Cameron JL, Geschwind JF, et al. Liver- Directed Therapy for Hepatic Metastases in Patients Undergoing Pancreaticoduodenectomy: A DualCenter Analysis. Annals of Surgery. Jul 2010;252(1):142-8.

123. Le Treut YP, Grégoire E, Klempnauer J, Belghiti J, Jouve E, Lerut J, et al. Liver Transplantation for Neuroendocrine Tumors in Europe-Results and Trends in Patient Selection: A 213-Case European Liver Transplant Registry Study. Annals of Surgery. May 2013;257(5):807-15.

124. Falconi M, Bartsch DK, Eriksson B, Kloppel G, Lopes JM, O'Connor JM, et al. ENETS Consensus Guidelines for the Management of Patients with Digestive Neuroendocrine Neoplasms of the Digestive System: Well-Differentiated Pancreatic Non-Functioning Tumors. Neuroendocrinology. 2012;95(2):120-34.

125. Shamiyeh A. Laparoscopic resection of gastrointestinal neuroendocrine tumors with special contribution of radionuclide imaging. WJG. 2014;20(42):15608.

126. Delbaldo C, Faivre S, Dreyer C, Raymond E. Sunitinib in advanced pancreatic neuroendocrine tumors: latest evidence and clinical potential. Ther Adv Med Oncol. Jan 2012;4(1):9-18.

127. Assarzadegan N, Montgomery E. What is New in the 2019 World Health Organization (WHO) Classification of Tumors of the Digestive System: Review of Selected Updates on Neuroendocrine Neoplasms, Appendiceal Tumors, and Molecular Testing. Archives of Pathology & Laboratory Medicine. June 1, 2021;145(6):664-77.

128. Hu X, Li D, Wang R, Wang P, Cai J. Comparison of the application of 18F-FDG and 68Ga-DOTATATE PET/CT in neuroendocrine tumors: A retrospective study. Medicine. May 12, 2023;102(19):e33726.

129. Adnan A, Basu S. Somatostatin Receptor Targeted PET-CT and Its Role in the Management and Theranostics of Gastroenteropancreatic Neuroendocrine Neoplasms. Diagnostics. June 24, 2023;13(13):2154.

130. Harris PE, Zhernosekov K. The evolution of PRRT for the treatment of neuroendocrine tumors; What comes next? Front Endocrinol. Oct 31, 2022;13:941832.

131. Hofland J, Brabander T, Verburg FA, Feelders RA, De Herder WW. Peptide Receptor Radionuclide Therapy. The Journal of Clinical Endocrinology & Metabolism. 25 Nov 2022;107(12):3199-208.

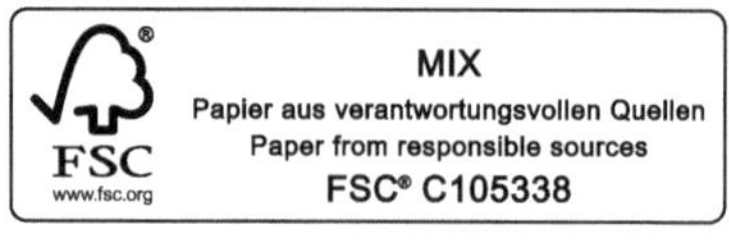

Printed by Books on Demand GmbH, Norderstedt / Germany